DASH DIET MEAL PREP CONTAINER

BY

JOANN K. LESLIE

Copyright © 2023 by Joann K. Leslie

ABOUT THE AUTHOR

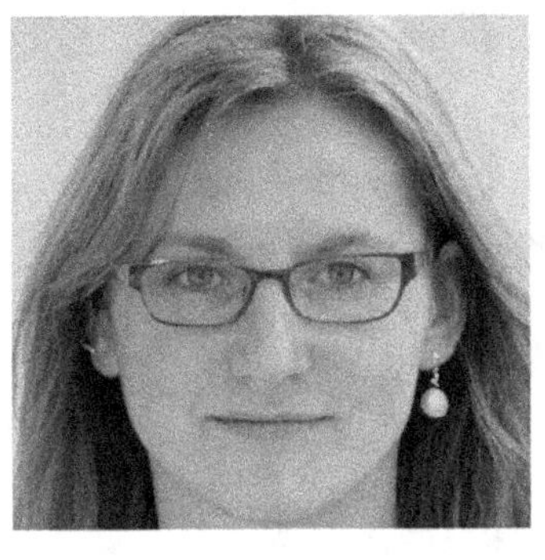 Step into the realm of culinary enchantment with Joann K. Leslie, a celebrated cook and luminary in the world of cookbooks, foods and wine. Joann's journey, like the sizzle of a well-seasoned pan, began in bustling kitchens and vineyards, fueled by an insatiable curiosity for the culinary arts.

Her pen, akin to the deft hands of a skilled chef, slices through the complexities of gastronomy, revealing the essence of ingredients and the transformative magic that turns meals into celebrations. Beyond mere instruction, Joann's writing is an exploration of culture, tradition, and the artistry that turns each dish into a unique narrative, waiting to be savored.

Joann's cookbooks serve as guides, encouraging readers to elevate their culinary skills and infuse creativity into their kitchen endeavors. The cultural odyssey we touched upon finds its echo in Joann's writing, where she unfolds the diverse tapestry of global cuisines with every turn of the page.

Mirroring the joy of fast and flavorful Dash Diet meals, Joann's focus on nutritious ingredients and mindful cooking techniques promotes a balanced and healthful approach to eating. Her recipes ensure that readers savor not only delicious flavors but also well-being.

Joann's writings transform every dining experience into a moment of joy. Whether shared with loved ones or savored in solitude, each meal becomes a chapter in a larger story.

Joann K. Leslie invites you on a journey where each page turns into a culinary adventure, and every recipe becomes a cherished memory.

BONUS PAGE

DASH DIET DELIGHTS: 15-MINUTE MEAL JAR

Welcome to the world of Dash Diet Delights! In this bonus section, we're diving into the exhilarating realm of fast and flavorful meals that not only align with the principles of the Dash Diet but also make your taste buds dance with joy. Say goodbye to lengthy meal preparations and hello to the sheer delight of savoring wholesome goodness in every bite, all within the span of 15 minutes. Let's embark on a culinary journey where speed meets satisfaction, proving that eating healthy can be an absolute delight!

Prepare to elevate your Dash Diet experience by exploring the art of assembling vibrant and nutritious meals – all within the trendy confines of a mason jar! These delightful, portable creations not only pack a nutritional punch but also serve as a canvas for your culinary creativity. Discover the joy of layering fresh ingredients, creating visually stunning combinations, and enjoying the convenience of meals that are as Instagram-worthy as they are delicious. Join us as we unlock the secrets of jarred cuisine, transforming your dining experience into a symphony of colors, textures, and flavors.

THREE LIGHTNING-FAST RECIPES DESIGNED FOR JAR CONVENIENCE

Here are the ingredients and preparation steps for each recipe without specifying layers:

1. MEDITERRANEAN QUINOA BLISS

INGREDIENTS:

Cooked quinoa, Cherry tomatoes, Cucumber, Red onion, Feta cheese, Kalamata olives, Balsamic glaze.

PREPARATION:

- Combine cooked quinoa, cherry tomatoes, cucumber, and red onion in a mixing bowl.
- Add crumbled feta cheese and Kalamata olives.
- Drizzle with balsamic glaze.

2. TROPICAL CHICKEN PARADISE:

INGREDIENTS:

Grilled chicken breast, Pineapple chunks, Mango slices, Red bell pepper, Yellow bell pepper,

Shredded coconut, Chopped cilantro, Lime vinaigrette.

PREPARATION:

- Mix grilled chicken breast, pineapple chunks, mango slices, and sliced bell peppers.
- Sprinkle shredded coconut and chopped cilantro.
- Top with lime vinaigrette.

3. POWER-PACKED VEGGIE CRUNCH:

INGREDIENTS:

Hummus or Greek yogurt, Cherry tomatoes, Cucumber, Bell peppers, Avocado, Broccoli florets, Mixed nuts and seeds, Olive oil, Herbs.

PREPARATION:

- Spread hummus or Greek yogurt at the base.
- Combine cherry tomatoes, cucumber, and bell peppers.
- Add avocado slices and steamed broccoli florets.
- Top with mixed nuts and seeds.
- Drizzle with olive oil and sprinkle herbs.

Feel free to adapt these recipes according to your preferences and dietary needs!

CREATIVE SUGGESTIONS FOR MIXING AND MATCHING INGREDIENTS FOR ENDLESS VARIETY

Here are some creative suggestions for mixing and matching ingredients to add endless variety to your jarred meals:

- **Global Fusion:** Mix and match ingredients from different cuisines to create a fusion of flavors. Combine quinoa, black beans, corn, salsa, and avocado for a Mexican-inspired jar, or try brown rice, teriyaki chicken, broccoli, and sesame seeds for an Asian twist.

- **Colorful Rainbow Jars:** Create visually appealing jars by incorporating a variety of colorful fruits and vegetables. Think red peppers, orange carrots, yellow corn, green spinach, blueberries, and purple cabbage for a vibrant and nutrient-packed meal.

- **Protein Power Play:** Experiment with different protein sources to keep things interesting. Swap grilled chicken with chickpeas, tofu, or shrimp. Consider adding hard-boiled eggs, quinoa, or edamame for a protein boost.

- **Seasonal Surprises:** Embrace seasonal produce for freshness and variety. In the summer, use tomatoes, basil, and fresh mozzarella. In the fall, incorporate roasted butternut squash, apples, and pecans for a cozy feel.

- **Textural Harmony:** Pay attention to textures to enhance the eating experience. Combine crunchy elements like nuts or seeds with creamy ones like avocado or feta. Include both raw and roasted veggies for a satisfying mix of textures.

- **Herbs and Spices Extravaganza:** Elevate your jars with a variety of herbs and spices. Add fresh basil, cilantro, mint, or dill for an herbal kick. Experiment with spices like cumin, paprika, or curry powder to infuse bold flavors.

- **Grains Galore:** Don't limit yourself to just one grain. Mix quinoa with farro, brown rice with barley, or couscous with bulgur for a diverse and hearty base.

- **Dress it Up:** Experiment with different dressings and sauces to transform your jarred creations. Try a zesty citrus vinaigrette, a tahini drizzle, or a creamy avocado dressing for added flavor.

- **Cheese Combinations:** Play with different cheeses to add richness. Feta pairs well with Mediterranean flavors, while goat cheese complements berries and nuts. Cheddar or gouda can add depth to roasted vegetables.

- **Leftover Remix:** Use leftovers creatively. If you had grilled vegetables or roasted chicken for dinner, repurpose them into a delicious jarred lunch the next day.

Mixing and matching these ingredients will not only provide endless variety but also keep your jarred meals exciting and enjoyable. Feel free to tailor these suggestions to your taste preferences and dietary needs!

TABLE OF CONTENTS

INTRODUCTION

In a bustling city where time was a precious commodity, Joann K. Leslie discovered a secret weapon for maintaining a healthy lifestyle—her Dash Diet meal prep container. Juggling work, family, and fitness, she realized the transformative power of this compact marvel. With compartments designed for mindful portions, the container became **Joann K. Leslie's** ally in crafting balanced, nutritious meals on the go.

Every morning, she filled the container with vibrant vegetables, lean proteins, and wholesome grains. The magic unfolded during lunchtime when, amidst meetings and deadlines, Joann K. Leslie unveiled her personalized culinary masterpiece. The Dash Diet container not only preserved the freshness of each ingredient but also encouraged mindful eating, making every bite a celebration of health.

Weeks passed, and Joann K. Leslie revealed newfound energy and vitality. Her Dash Diet container became a symbol of empowerment, enabling her to make conscious food choices amid life's chaos. The benefits reverberated beyond personal well-being; Joann K. Leslie inspired colleagues to join the healthy living revolution, creating a ripple effect of positive change.

As the sun set on another hectic day, Joann K. Leslie marveled at the impact of a simple container on her journey to a healthier life. It wasn't just a vessel; it was a catalyst for a transformative lifestyle, proving that, in the midst of life's whirlwind, a Dash Diet meal prep container could be the anchor to sustained health and wellness.

CHAPTER 1

DASH DIET

The meaning of DASH is "Dietary Approaches to Stop Hypertension." It aims at controlling high blood pressure, or hypertension through a specific dietary regimen. The program advocates for the consumption of wholesome foods that benefit health while also reducing salt intake. Achieving and maintaining balance marks the ultimate goal in promoting heart-healthy eating habits via this plan.

The DASH diet is characterized by remarkable attributes such as:

- The DASH diet gives importance to fruits and vegetables due to their abundant supply of vitamins, minerals, and antioxidants.

- In order to encourage a wholesome diet, it is advisable to advocate the consumption of lean sources of protein like poultry, fish, nuts and beans. On the other hand, limit the intake of red meat and processed meats.

- Opt for whole grains such as brown rice, oats and whole wheat instead of refined types to acquire greater amounts of fiber and nutrients.

- Choosing dairy products with low fat or no fat is recommended by experts as they contain high amounts of calcium and protein.

- To maintain a healthy heart, it is recommended to consume nuts, seeds and legumes due to their beneficial fats and nutritional value. Therefore, encouragement is offered towards incorporating these foods in your diet.

- The emphasis of the DASH eating plan is on reducing sodium intake, as consuming excessive salt has been linked to an increase in blood pressure readings.

- It is recommended to practice moderation when eating sweets and foods containing added sugars.

Several researches have established the DASH diet to be effective in decreasing blood pressure and improving cardiovascular health, resulting in healthcare experts acknowledging it worldwide. This method of eating is not only advantageous for people with hypertension but also considered a wholesome dietary routine appropriate for everyone.

HEALTH BENEFITS OF DASH

In addition to its primary objective of managing blood pressure, the DASH (Dietary Approaches to Stop Hypertension) diet provides various other health benefits. A few significant advantages of this eating plan include:

- DASH is famous for its ability to significantly lower blood pressure, especially in those diagnosed with hypertension. This contributes greatly towards improving overall cardiovascular well-being.

- To maintain a healthy heart, it is important to prioritize consuming fruits, vegetables, lean proteins and whole grains. These food groups can help decrease the likelihood of developing heart disease and enhance cholesterol levels.

- The DASH program advocates for a well-balanced and nutrient-rich eating plan that not only helps with weight management but also lowers the chances of health problems associated with obesity.

- Enhanced Nutrient Consumption: By emphasizing the intake of nutrient-dense foods such as vitamins, minerals and antioxidants, this regimen promotes improved physical health.

- The DASH program's emphasis on consuming whole, unprocessed foods can decrease the likelihood of developing chronic illnesses including diabetes and certain types of cancer.

- Improved Kidney Function: By prioritizing a moderate consumption of protein and adopting wholesome dietary habits, this regime can fortify kidney well-being.

- In the management of diabetes, adhering to DASH principles is recommended as it promotes healthy eating habits and balanced carbohydrate intake.

- Elevated fiber consumption can be achieved by incorporating whole grains, fruits, and vegetables into the DASH diet. This results in improved digestive health for individuals as recommended levels of fiber are met.

- By promoting a decrease in sodium intake, the DASH program aids in preventing water retention and maintaining optimal blood pressure.

- DASH offers a viable and adjustable dietary strategy, rendering it an appropriate sustainable alternative for people striving to enhance their general wellbeing in the long run.

- By embracing the DASH diet, one can experience a myriad of advantageous health outcomes that improve overall wellness and diminish the likelihood of developing chronic ailments.

HOW DASH HELPS WITH HYPERTENSION

The DASH (Dietary Approaches to Stop Hypertension) diet is specifically designed to help manage and prevent hypertension (high blood pressure). Here's how the DASH diet contributes to hypertension management:

- Lower Sodium Intake: The DASH diet recommends reducing sodium intake, a key factor in hypertension. By limiting salt, the diet helps prevent fluid retention and decreases blood pressure.

- Rich in Potassium, Calcium, and Magnesium: The DASH diet emphasizes foods rich in potassium, calcium, and magnesium. These minerals play roles in blood pressure regulation, contributing to overall cardiovascular health.

- Balanced Nutrition: The diet encourages a balanced and varied intake of nutrient-dense foods, including fruits, vegetables, lean proteins, and whole grains. This balanced approach supports overall health and may positively impact blood pressure.

- Increased Fiber Intake: Whole grains, fruits, and vegetables included in the DASH diet are excellent sources of dietary fiber. Higher fiber intake is associated with lower blood pressure and improved heart health.

- Moderate Alcohol Consumption: The DASH diet recommends moderate alcohol consumption, which has been associated with certain heart health benefits. However, it's crucial to adhere to recommended limits to avoid adverse effects on blood pressure.

- Limiting Saturated and Trans Fats: The DASH diet encourages the consumption of healthy fats while limiting saturated and trans fats. This can positively impact cholesterol levels and contribute to better cardiovascular health.

- Weight Management: Following the DASH diet can contribute to weight management or weight loss, which is often beneficial for individuals with hypertension. Maintaining a healthy weight is linked to lower blood pressure.

- Lifestyle Integration: The DASH diet is not just about food; it also emphasizes lifestyle factors like regular physical activity. Exercise complements dietary changes, promoting overall cardiovascular health and blood pressure control.

- Scientifically Supported: Numerous studies have demonstrated the effectiveness of the DASH diet in reducing blood pressure. Its evidence-based approach makes it a recommended dietary strategy for those with hypertension.

- Long-Term Health Benefits: Beyond immediate blood pressure reduction, the DASH diet's focus on a balanced and nutritious eating pattern contributes to long-term health benefits, reducing the risk of cardiovascular diseases associated with hypertension.

By incorporating these principles, the DASH diet provides a comprehensive and sustainable approach to managing hypertension. As always, individuals with specific health concerns should consult with healthcare professionals for personalized advice and guidance.

HOW DASH HELPS WITH WEIGHT LOSS

The DASH (Dietary Approaches to Stop Hypertension) diet is not designed specifically for weight loss, but its principles can support weight management. Here's how the DASH diet can contribute to weight loss:

- Emphasis on Nutrient-Dense Foods: The DASH diet encourages the consumption of nutrient-dense foods, such as fruits, vegetables, lean proteins, and whole grains. These foods are generally lower in calories while providing essential nutrients, making them a smart choice for weight management.

- Portion Control: The DASH diet promotes portion control, which is crucial for managing caloric intake. By being mindful of portion sizes, individuals can reduce overall calorie consumption, aiding in weight loss.

- Lower Sodium Intake: Reduced sodium intake helps prevent water retention and bloating. While not contributing directly to fat loss, it can influence the perception of body weight and contribute to a healthier overall appearance.

- Balanced Macronutrients: The DASH diet encourages a balanced intake of macronutrients, including carbohydrates, proteins, and fats. This balance can help regulate hunger and promote satiety, making it easier to maintain a calorie deficit for weight loss.

- Higher Fiber Intake: The DASH diet includes a variety of high-fiber foods, such as fruits, vegetables, and whole grains. High-fiber foods are more filling, which can help control appetite and reduce overall food intake.

- Limitation of Processed Foods: The DASH diet recommends minimizing processed and refined foods, which are often high in added sugars and unhealthy fats. By avoiding these types of foods, individuals can reduce their overall calorie and sugar intake, supporting weight loss.

- Encouragement of Healthy Fats: While the DASH diet limits saturated and trans fats, it encourages the consumption of healthy fats from sources like olive oil, avocados, and nuts. Including these fats can contribute to satiety and flavor, making meals more satisfying.

- Lifestyle Recommendations: The DASH diet is not only about food but also includes recommendations for a healthy lifestyle, such as regular physical activity. Exercise is a key component of any successful weight loss plan.

- Scientific Support: Studies have suggested that following the DASH diet may result in weight loss, particularly when combined with a calorie-controlled diet and increased physical activity.

While the primary goal of the DASH diet is to manage blood pressure, its emphasis on whole, nutrient-dense foods and healthy lifestyle habits can align with general principles of weight management. Individuals looking to lose weight should consult with healthcare professionals or registered dietitians for personalized advice and guidance.

MAKING THE DASH DIET FIT YOUR LIFESTYLE

Adapting the DASH (Dietary Approaches to Stop Hypertension) diet to fit your lifestyle can be a rewarding and sustainable approach. Here are some tips to make the DASH diet work seamlessly with your daily routine:

- Gradual Transition: Start by making small, gradual changes to your eating habits. This allows you to adjust without feeling overwhelmed.

- Identify Personal Preferences: Tailor the DASH diet to your taste preferences. Identify your favorite fruits, vegetables, lean proteins, and whole grains to create meals you genuinely enjoy.

- Meal Planning and Prep: Plan your meals and snacks ahead of time. This helps you make thoughtful choices and reduces the temptation to opt for less healthy options on a whim.

- Customize Recipes: Modify DASH-friendly recipes to suit your preferences. Experiment with different herbs, spices, and cooking methods to add variety and flavor.

- Flexible Eating Patterns: The DASH diet is adaptable. Whether you prefer three larger meals or several smaller ones, find an eating pattern that aligns with your lifestyle and keeps you satisfied.

- Smart Swaps: Make smart food substitutions. For example, replace refined grains with whole grains, choose lean proteins, and opt for healthy fats like olive oil.

- Portable Snacks: Keep portable, DASH-friendly snacks on hand. This helps you avoid unhealthy choices when you're on the go.

- Social Eating: Navigate social situations by making informed choices. Choose DASH-friendly options when dining out and communicate your dietary preferences to friends and family.

- Mindful Eating: Practice mindful eating. Pay attention to hunger and fullness cues, savor your food, and eat without distractions to foster a positive relationship with food.

- Hydration: Stay hydrated with water. Limit sugary drinks and be mindful of alcohol intake. Hydration is an essential aspect of the DASH diet.

- Smart Shopping: When grocery shopping, stick to the perimeter of the store where fresh produce, lean proteins, and whole grains are often located. Read labels to check for added sugars and sodium.

- Physical Activity: Incorporate regular physical activity into your routine. Exercise complements the DASH diet for overall health and well-being.

- Seek Support: Share your DASH journey with friends or family members. Having a support system can make it easier to stay on track and share recipe ideas.

- Flexibility on Occasions: Allow for flexibility on special occasions. It's okay to enjoy treats occasionally, as long as you balance them with overall healthy eating.

Remember, the DASH diet is adaptable and can be customized to suit individual preferences and lifestyles. Finding joy in the foods you eat and making sustainable changes over time are key to successfully incorporating the DASH principles into your daily routine.

DASH DIET GUIDELINES

The DASH (Dietary Approaches to Stop Hypertension) diet provides specific guidelines to help individuals manage and prevent high blood pressure.

Here are the key principles and guidelines of the DASH diet:

DAILY SERVINGS OF DIFFERENT FOOD GROUPS

- **Vegetables:** Aim for 4-5 servings per day.
- **Fruits:** Target 4-5 servings per day.
- **Grains:** Choose whole grains and aim for 6-8 servings per day.
- **Lean Proteins:** Include 2 or fewer servings of lean meat, poultry, or fish daily.
- **Nuts, Seeds, and Legumes:** Consume 4-5 servings per week.
- **Dairy:** Choose low-fat or fat-free options and aim for 2 or fewer servings daily.
- **Sodium Intake:** Limit sodium to 2,300 milligrams per day for a standard DASH diet. For an even lower sodium version, aim for 1,500 milligrams per day.
- **Fats and Oils:** Opt for healthy fats, such as olive oil and nuts, in moderation. Limit saturated fat and total fat intake.

DASH EATING PLAN

Follow the DASH eating plan, which includes a variety of foods from all food groups while emphasizing fruits, vegetables, and low-fat dairy.

PORTION CONTROL

Be mindful of portion sizes to maintain a healthy calorie balance.

ALCOHOL MODERATION

If you consume alcohol, do so in moderation. For women, this means up to one drink per day, and for men, up to two drinks per day.

PHYSICAL ACTIVITY

Incorporate regular physical activity into your routine for overall health benefits.

NUTRIENT-RICH CHOICES

Choose nutrient-dense foods to ensure you get a variety of essential vitamins and minerals.

GRADUAL CHANGES

Make dietary changes gradually to allow for easier adaptation to the DASH diet.

CONSULTATION WITH HEALTHCARE PROVIDER

Before making significant dietary changes, especially for those with existing health conditions, consult with a healthcare provider.

By following these guidelines, individuals can adopt the DASH diet as a sustainable and effective approach to promote heart health, manage blood pressure, and improve overall well-being.

WHAT TO EAT ON THE DASH DIET

- **Fruits and Vegetables:** Aim for a range of promising fruits and veggies. They are high in important vitamins, minerals, and antioxidants.

- **Whole Grains:** Choose whole grains like brown rice, quinoa, oats, and whole wheat for fiber and nutrients.

- **Lean Proteins:** Opt for lean protein sources such as poultry, fish, beans, lentils, tofu, and nuts.

- **Dairy:** Select low-fat or fat-free dairy products for calcium and protein without excessive saturated fat.

- **Nuts, Seeds, and Legumes:** Incorporate nuts, seeds, and legumes for healthy fats, protein, and fiber.

- **Healthy Fats:** Include sources of healthy fats, such as olive oil, avocados, and fatty fish like salmon.

- **Low-Sodium Foods:** Choose foods with lower sodium content and use herbs and spices for flavoring.

- **Limited Sweets:** Consume sweets and added sugars in moderation.

- **Portion Control:** Be mindful of portion sizes to maintain a healthy calorie balance.

- **Hydration:** Stay well-hydrated with water and limit sugary beverages.

WHAT TO LIMIT OR AVOID ON THE DASH DIET

- **High-Sodium Foods:** Minimize the intake of high-sodium foods, including processed and packaged foods.

- **Processed Meats:** Limit processed meats such as bacon, sausage, and deli meats, which can be high in sodium and saturated fats.

- **High-Fat Dairy:** Reduce consumption of high-fat dairy products, opting for low-fat or fat-free alternatives.

- **Sweets and Added Sugars:** Limit the intake of sweets, sugary beverages, and foods high in added sugars.

- **Saturated and Trans Fats:** Cut back on foods high in saturated and trans fats, like fried foods and commercially baked goods.

- **Excessive Alcohol:** Consume alcohol in moderation, if at all.

- **Caffeine:** While not strictly restricted, excessive caffeine intake may be limited for some individuals.

Remember, the DASH diet is flexible and can be adapted based on individual preferences and dietary needs. It's always advisable to consult with a healthcare professional or a registered dietitian when making significant changes to your diet, especially if you have underlying health conditions.

CHAPTER 2

BASICS OF MEAL PREPPING

Meal prepping is a practical and efficient approach to preparing and organizing meals in advance. Here are the basics of meal prepping:

- Planning: Begin by organizing your weekly menu. Take into account your schedule, food choices, and nutritional requirements.

- Choose Balanced Recipes: Select recipes that include a variety of nutrient-dense foods, such as lean proteins, whole grains, fruits, and vegetables.

- Make a Shopping List: Based on your chosen recipes, create a shopping list. This helps streamline grocery shopping and ensures you have all the necessary ingredients.

- Batch Cooking: Prepare ingredients in larger quantities to create multiple servings. Batch cooking saves time and ensures consistency in portion sizes.

- Storage Containers: Invest in a variety of reusable storage containers. Choose containers with compartments to keep different food items separate and maintain freshness.

- Portion Control: Portion meals according to your nutritional needs. This helps with calorie control and ensures a balanced intake of nutrients.

- Labeling: Label containers with the date of preparation to keep track of freshness. This is especially crucial when it comes to perishable goods.

- Refrigeration and Freezing: Refrigerate meals for consumption within a few days. For longer storage, consider freezing meals and reheating them as needed.

- Diverse Ingredients: Use a variety of ingredients to keep your meals interesting and ensure you receive a broad spectrum of nutrients.

- Prep Snacks: Extend meal prepping to snacks. Prepare healthy snacks like cut vegetables, fruit slices, or yogurt cups to have convenient and nutritious options readily available.

- Adaptability: Be flexible and adaptable. You don't need to prep every meal for the entire week; even prepping a few meals or key ingredients can make a significant difference.

- Mindful Eating: Use meal prepping as an opportunity for mindful eating. Pay attention to portion sizes, savor the flavors, and enjoy the convenience of having nutritious meals readily available.

- Consistency: Aim for consistency in your meal prepping routine. Whether it's a weekly or bi-weekly practice, regularity makes it easier to maintain a healthy eating pattern.

Meal prepping not only saves time but also encourages healthier food choices by eliminating the need for last-minute, potentially less nutritious options. Whether you're focused on weight management, dietary goals, or simply seeking convenience, mastering the basics of meal prepping can make a positive impact on your overall well-being.

WHAT MEAL PREP IS (AND WHY IT WORKS WELL WITH DASH)

Meal prep involves planning, preparing, and portioning meals ahead of time to make eating healthier, more convenient, and efficient. It aligns seamlessly with the principles of the DASH (Dietary Approaches to Stop Hypertension) diet for several reasons:

- Portion Control: Meal prepping allows you to control portion sizes, a key element in the DASH diet. Precise portions help manage calorie intake and ensure a balanced distribution of nutrients.

- Nutrient-Rich Choices: Planning meals in advance facilitates the inclusion of a variety of nutrient-dense foods, such as fruits, vegetables, lean proteins, and whole grains, as recommended by the DASH diet.

- Reduced Sodium Intake: By preparing meals at home, you have better control over the ingredients, helping you limit the use of high-sodium additives commonly found in processed and restaurant foods.

- Consistency: Meal prepping promotes consistency in adhering to the DASH diet. Having pre-prepared, healthy meals readily available reduces the likelihood of resorting to less nutritious options on busy days.

- Time Efficiency: DASH-friendly meal prepping saves time during busy weekdays. It streamlines the cooking process, making it easier to incorporate a variety of nutrient-rich foods into your daily meals.

- Encourages Balanced Eating: Planning meals in advance encourages a well-balanced approach to eating, meeting the DASH diet's emphasis on a mix of fruits, vegetables, lean proteins, and whole grains.

- Reduces Decision Fatigue: Knowing what you'll eat in advance eliminates the need to make spontaneous, potentially less healthy choices when hunger strikes. This aligns with the DASH diet's focus on mindful and intentional eating.

- Cost-Effective: Meal prepping can be cost-effective, as you can buy ingredients in bulk, reducing the reliance on convenience foods that may be pricier and less aligned with DASH diet principles.

- Customization: Tailoring your meal prep to your taste preferences and dietary needs ensures that you enjoy your food, making it more likely that you'll stick to the DASH diet in the long run.

- Long-Term Sustainability: The convenience and structure of meal prepping make it a sustainable approach to healthy eating, supporting the long-term goals of the DASH diet for heart health and overall well-being.

In summary, meal prep enhances the effectiveness of the DASH diet by promoting consistency, providing control over ingredients, and streamlining the process of incorporating DASH-friendly foods into your daily routine.

WHY PREP

Meal prepping offers several compelling reasons, often abbreviated as the acronym PREP, to encourage individuals to plan, prepare, and organize their meals in advance:

- Planning for Success: Meal prepping allows you to plan your meals strategically, helping you make healthier food choices and stay on track with your dietary goals.

- Reclaiming Time: By dedicating a specific time for meal preparation, you reclaim time during the week. This helps reduce the stress and time constraints associated with daily meal decisions.

- Efficiency in Execution: Preparing meals in batches is efficient and time-saving. It streamlines the cooking process, making it easier to manage your overall schedule.

- Portion Control: Meal prepping facilitates portion control, a crucial element for weight management and overall health. It helps avoid overeating and promotes balanced nutrition.

These four key points encapsulate the "PREP" concept, highlighting the benefits of planning and preparing meals ahead of time. Whether you're focusing on health, convenience, or time management, meal prepping emerges as a valuable strategy for fostering positive eating habits and enhancing overall well-being.

MEAL PREP GUIDELINES (STEPS TO SUCCESSFUL MEAL PREP)

Successful meal prep involves a systematic approach to planning, preparing, and organizing meals ahead of time. Here are step-by-step guidelines for effective meal prep:

- Set Clear Goals: Define your meal prep goals, whether it's saving time, managing portions, or aligning with specific dietary needs.

- Plan Your Meals: Create a weekly or bi-weekly meal plan that includes a variety of nutrient-dense foods. Consider your nutritional requirements and taste preferences.

- Make a Shopping List: Using your meal plan as a guide, make a thorough list of everything you need to buy.

- Choose a Prep Day: Designate a specific day or two for meal prep. This could be a weekend or a day when you have more time available.

- Batch Cooking: Cook larger quantities of proteins, grains, and vegetables in batches. This streamlines the cooking process and ensures you have pre-prepared components for meals.

- Use Quality Storage Containers: Invest in good-quality, airtight storage containers with compartments. This helps keep different food items separate and maintains freshness.

- Portion Control: Practice portion control when dividing meals into containers. This helps manage calorie intake and ensures a balanced distribution of nutrients.

- Labeling: Label containers with the date of preparation to keep track of freshness. Use labels to identify specific meals and ingredients.

- Refrigeration and Freezing: Refrigerate meals that will be consumed within a few days. Freeze portions for longer storage. Ensure proper thawing before reheating.

- Diverse Ingredients: Incorporate a variety of ingredients to keep your meals interesting and nutritionally diverse.

- Prep Snacks: Extend meal prepping to snacks. Prepare healthy snack options like cut vegetables, fruit slices, or yogurt cups.

- Mindful Eating: Practice mindful eating by paying attention to portion sizes, savoring the flavors, and eating without distractions.

- Consistency: Establish a consistent meal prep routine. Regularity makes it easier to maintain healthy eating habits over the long term.

- Adaptability: Be adaptable and open to adjusting your meal prep plan based on your evolving needs and preferences.

- Store Cooked and Raw Separately: When prepping ingredients, store cooked and raw items separately to maintain food safety and prevent cross-contamination.

- Easy-to-Assemble Meals: Prepare components that can be easily assembled into complete meals later. This adds flexibility to your eating routine.

- Reuse Ingredients: Plan meals that utilize common ingredients to minimize waste and make shopping more efficient.

- Enjoy the Process: Approach meal prep as a positive and enjoyable activity. Experiment with new recipes and cooking techniques to keep it interesting.

By following these guidelines, you can streamline your meal prep process, save time, and ensure that you have healthy, delicious meals readily available throughout the week.

CHAPTER 3

CREATING YOUR DASH KITCHEN

Creating a DASH (Dietary Approaches to Stop Hypertension) kitchen involves setting up your culinary space to align with the principles of the DASH diet. Here's a guide to help you create a DASH kitchen:

1. Stock up on Fresh Produce
Purpose: The DASH diet emphasizes fruits and vegetables. Ensure your kitchen is always stocked with a variety of fresh produce to incorporate into your meals.

2. Whole Grains Galore
Purpose: Choose whole grains such as brown rice, quinoa, oats, and whole wheat pasta. These provide fiber and nutrients crucial for heart health.

3. Lean Proteins
Purpose: Opt for lean protein sources like poultry, fish, beans, and legumes. Keep your freezer stocked with these options for easy access.

4. Healthy Fats

Purpose: Include sources of healthy fats such as olive oil, avocados, and nuts. These contribute to overall heart health and add flavor to your meals.

5. Low-Fat Dairy

Purpose: Choose low-fat or fat-free dairy products, such as milk, yogurt, and cheese. These supply vital nutrients without having too many saturated fats.

6. Herbs and Spices

Purpose: DASH meals are flavorful without excessive salt. Stock your pantry with a variety of herbs, spices, and seasoning blends to enhance taste without compromising on health.

7. Food Labels and Nutrition Education

Purpose: Familiarize yourself with reading food labels to identify sodium content. Stay informed about nutritional values to make healthier choices.

8. Meal Prep Containers

Purpose: Prepare and store DASH-friendly meals in advance using portion-controlled containers. This encourages mindful eating and prevents over-consumption.

9. Quality Knives and Cutting Boards

Purpose: Make chopping and preparing fruits and vegetables a breeze with quality knives and cutting boards. Efficient preparation encourages the consumption of fresh produce.

10. Digital Kitchen Scale

Purpose: Weighing ingredients helps with portion control. This is particularly important for grains, proteins, and other components of your DASH meals.

11. Non-Stick Cookware

Purpose: Use non-stick pans to minimize the need for excessive cooking oils. This aligns with the DASH diet's focus on healthy fats.

12. Baking Sheets and Pans

Purpose: Roast vegetables or lean proteins on baking sheets for easy and healthy meal preparation.

13. DASH-Friendly Cookbooks

Purpose: Explore recipes specifically designed for the DASH diet. This ensures variety and creativity in your meals while adhering to dietary guidelines.

14. Educational Resources

Purpose: Stay informed about the DASH diet through books, articles, and reputable online resources. Understanding the principles helps you make informed choices.

15. Hydration Station

Purpose: Keep a water filter or water bottles easily accessible. Staying hydrated is an integral part of the DASH diet.

16. Mindful Eating Space

Purpose: Create a comfortable and mindful eating space. Turn off distractions, savor your meals, and pay attention to hunger and fullness cues.

17. DASH Diet App or Journal

Purpose: Use a DASH diet app or journal to track your daily food intake, ensuring you meet nutritional goals and stay on track.

18. Herb Garden

Purpose: If possible, cultivate a small herb garden. Fresh herbs add depth to your dishes without the need for excess salt.

19. Educational Posters or Visual Aids

Purpose: Hang posters or visual aids in your kitchen that display DASH-friendly foods and serving sizes. This serves as a constant reminder of your dietary goals.

20. Regular Grocery Shopping Routine
Purpose: Establish a regular grocery shopping routine to ensure your kitchen is consistently stocked with fresh and wholesome ingredients.

Creating a DASH kitchen involves a combination of mindful food choices, strategic organization, and culinary education. By setting up your kitchen with the principles of the DASH diet in mind, you create an environment that supports your journey toward better heart health and overall well-being.

TIPS FOR GROCERY SHOPPING

Efficient and mindful grocery shopping is crucial for successful meal prep and maintaining a healthy diet. Here are some tips for making the most of your grocery shopping experience:

- Plan Before You Go: Make a meal plan for the week and create a corresponding shopping list. This helps you stay focused and reduces the likelihood of impulse purchases.

- Shop the Perimeter: The perimeter of the grocery store typically houses fresh produce, lean proteins, dairy, and whole grains. Focus on these areas for the majority of your shopping.

- Prioritize Fresh Produce: Load up on a variety of fruits and vegetables. Choose seasonal produce for freshness and cost-effectiveness.

- Read Labels: Check nutrition labels for information on ingredients, added sugars, and sodium content. Opt for products with minimal processing.

- Choose Whole Grains: Select whole grains such as brown rice, quinoa, and whole wheat bread over refined grains. These provide more fiber and nutrients.

- Lean Proteins: Include lean protein sources like poultry, fish, beans, and tofu. Look for sales or discounts on proteins to save money.

- Options for Dairy: Select plant-based substitutes or dairy products with reduced or no fat.

- Healthy Fats: Pick up sources of healthy fats such as avocados, nuts, seeds, and olive oil.

- Frozen Produce: Stock up on frozen fruits and vegetables. They have a longer shelf life and are equally nutritious as fresh options.

- Limit Processed Foods: Minimize the purchase of processed and packaged foods, as they often contain added sugars, unhealthy fats, and preservatives.

- Mindful Snacking: If you buy snacks, choose healthier options like nuts, seeds, or whole-grain crackers. Portion them into snack-sized bags for convenience.

- Buy in Bulk: Purchase non-perishable items in bulk, like grains, nuts, and legumes, to save money in the long run.

- Look for Sales and Discounts: Don't miss out on any discounts or sales.

- Use a Shopping Basket: Opt for a shopping basket instead of a cart for smaller trips. It helps prevent unnecessary purchases and encourages mindful shopping.

- Shop Alone: If possible, shop alone to minimize distractions and stick to your planned purchases.

- Bring Reusable Bags: Bring reusable bags to reduce plastic waste and, in some places, save on bag fees.

- Compare Prices: Compare prices and consider store brands, which are often more budget-friendly.

- Stick to Your List: Stay disciplined and stick to your shopping list. This helps prevent impulse buying.

- Be Wary of "Healthy" Labels: Some products labeled as "healthy" may still be high in sugar or other additives. Read labels carefully.

- Stay Hydrated: Drink water before and during your shopping trip to stay hydrated and avoid shopping while hungry.

By incorporating these tips into your grocery shopping routine, you can make healthier choices, save money, and streamline the process of preparing nutritious meals at home.

HELPFUL TOOLS FOR MEAL PREPPING AND THEIR USES

1. Quality Knife Set

Uses: A sharp knife set is indispensable for precision cutting, chopping, and dicing vegetables, fruits, and proteins. Different blade types allow for versatility in meal prep tasks, from slicing through delicate herbs to breaking down tougher cuts of meat.

2. Cutting Boards

Uses: Multiple cutting boards serve as dedicated surfaces for various food items, preventing cross-contamination. Use wood for fruits and vegetables, plastic for proteins, and keep one exclusively for cooked foods to maintain food safety.

3. Food Processor

Uses: A food processor is a multitasking powerhouse. From chopping and pureeing to shredding and blending, it expedites the preparation of sauces, dips, and even helps create fine crumbs for crusts or coatings.

Blender

Uses: Blenders are perfect for creating smoothies, soups, and purees. They efficiently combine ingredients, ensuring a smooth and consistent texture for a variety of recipes, from breakfast to dinner.

4. Mandoline Slicer

Uses: This tool provides uniform slices for vegetables and fruits, enhancing the visual appeal of dishes. Adjusting the thickness allows for versatility in meal presentation and cooking times.

5. Vegetable Peeler

Uses: A vegetable peeler is a quick and efficient way to peel fruits and vegetables. It's particularly handy for thin strips of vegetables or creating decorative garnishes.

6. Microplane Grater

Uses: This tool finely grates ingredients like garlic, ginger, citrus zest, and hard cheeses. It adds concentrated flavors and textures to dishes without overpowering them.

7. Mixing Bowls:

Uses: Available in various sizes, mixing bowls are essential for combining ingredients, marinating proteins, and tossing salads. They are versatile and come in materials suitable for both mixing and serving.

8.   Measuring Cups and Spoons:
Uses: Precision is key in meal prep, and these tools ensure accurate measurements for ingredients. From liquids to dry goods, they contribute to consistent and reliable cooking.

9.   Digital Kitchen Scale:
Uses: Weighing ingredients provides an additional level of accuracy, especially when following specific recipes or managing portion sizes for health and fitness goals.

10. Baking Sheets and Pans:
Uses: Essential for roasting vegetables, proteins, and preparing sheet pan meals. Non-stick options or those lined with parchment paper simplify cleanup.

11. Silicone Baking Mats:
Uses: These mats offer a non-stick surface for baking and roasting, reducing the need for excessive oils and making cleanup a breeze.

12. Instant-Read Thermometer:
Uses: Ensures proteins are cooked to a safe temperature, preventing undercooking or overcooking. It's a crucial tool for food safety and achieving the desired doneness.

13. Slow Cooker or Instant Pot:
Uses: Ideal for set-and-forget meals, these appliances allow for hands-free cooking of stews, soups, grains, and proteins. They're time-efficient and yield flavorful results.

14. Steamer Basket:
Uses: Preserves the nutrients in vegetables while cooking them quickly. It's an excellent tool for maintaining the color, flavor, and nutritional value of fresh produce.

15. Glass Storage Containers:
Uses: Microwave-safe, oven-safe, and eco-friendly containers for storing prepped meals. They are durable and offer a clear view of the contents.

16. Plastic Meal Prep Containers:
Uses: These containers are designed for portioning and storing individual meals, helping with portion control and ensuring a balanced distribution of nutrients.

17. Resealable Plastic Bags:
Uses: Convenient for marinating proteins or storing prepped ingredients in the freezer. They are versatile and space-efficient for storing items in the refrigerator or pantry.

18. Lunch Bags or Insulated Containers:
Uses: These keep prepped meals fresh when on the go, maintaining optimal temperature and preventing spoilage.

19. Ice Cube Trays:
Uses: Perfect for freezing individual portions of sauces, stocks, or herbs. They offer portion control and reduce waste.

20. Food Labels:
Uses: Essential for organizing and identifying the contents and date of preparation. Labels help prevent confusion and ensure food safety.

21. Egg Slicer:
Uses: Creates uniform slices of hard-boiled eggs for salads or garnishes, adding texture and protein to various dishes.

22. Can Opener:
Uses: Opens canned goods like beans or tomatoes, providing convenience and access to pantry staples.

23. Colander or Strainer:
Uses: Drains pasta, grains, and washed vegetables efficiently, ensuring proper preparation and preventing excess moisture in dishes.

24. Funnel:
Uses: Facilitates the pouring of liquids into containers without spills, ensuring precision in measurements and reducing mess.

25. Thermal Lunch Bag:
Uses: Keeps meals warm or cold for extended periods, ideal for packed lunches at work or school.

26. Wok or Stir-Fry Pan:
Uses: Perfect for quick and healthy stir-fry meals, allowing for the rapid cooking of a variety of vegetables and proteins.

27. Herb Keeper:
Uses: Extends the freshness of herbs, reducing waste and ensuring the availability of flavorful ingredients.

28. Non-Stick Cooking Spray:
Uses: A low-calorie option for coating pans, ensuring easy release of food, and preventing sticking without excess oil.

29. Sous Vide Precision Cooker:
Uses: Ensures precise cooking temperatures for proteins, resulting in tender and flavorful dishes. It's a modern method for achieving restaurant-quality results at home.

Investing in these tools not only streamlines your meal prep process but also enhances the overall efficiency and enjoyment of your time in the kitchen. Each tool serves a unique purpose, contributing to the success of your culinary endeavors.

PREPARED MEALS AND INGREDIENTS: SAFE STORING METHODS

Ensuring the safe storage of ingredients and prepared meals is crucial for maintaining freshness, preventing foodborne illnesses, and maximizing the benefits of your meal prep efforts. Here are ways to safely store both ingredients and prepared meals:

SAFELY STORING INGREDIENTS

1. Refrigeration: Store perishable items like meat, dairy, and certain fruits and vegetables in the refrigerator to slow down bacterial growth.

2. Proper Temperature Zones: Keep the refrigerator temperature at or below 40°F (4°C) and the freezer at 0°F (-18°C) to maintain food safety.

3. Air-Tight Containers: Transfer opened packages or ingredients to air-tight containers to prevent contamination and maintain freshness.

4. Produce Storage Bags: Use produce storage bags with proper ventilation to extend the shelf life of fruits and vegetables.

5. Separation of Raw and Cooked Foods: Store raw meats separately from cooked foods to avoid cross-contamination. Place raw meats on lower shelves to prevent drips onto other items.

6. Labeling and Dating: Clearly label and date items in the refrigerator to track freshness and ensure timely consumption.

7. Utilize Crisper Drawers: Store fruits and vegetables in designated crisper drawers with humidity controls to optimize freshness.

8. Freezer Storage: Freeze items that won't be used within a few days to extend their shelf life. Use freezer-safe containers or bags, and remove excess air to prevent freezer burn.

9. Storage of Pantry Items: Keep pantry staples (dry goods, canned goods) in a cool, dark, and dry place to maintain quality. Seal opened packages tightly.

10. Rotate Stock: Practice the "first in, first out" (FIFO) method to use older items before newer ones, reducing the risk of spoilage.

SAFELY STORING PREPARED MEALS

1. Portion Control Containers: Use portion control containers to divide meals into appropriate serving sizes, aiding in calorie control and preventing overconsumption.

2. Refrigerate Promptly: Place prepared meals in the refrigerator within two hours of cooking to prevent bacteria growth. If the ambient temperature is high, reduce this time to one hour.

3. Cooling Rack: Allow hot dishes to cool on a rack before refrigerating. This prevents uneven cooling and maintains food quality.

4. Cover or Wrap Well: Cover or wrap meals tightly with plastic wrap, aluminum foil, or in air-tight containers to prevent moisture loss and protect against odors in the refrigerator.

5. Labeling: Properly label each container with the date of preparation and its contents. This helps in tracking freshness and avoiding confusion.

6. Freezing Prepared Meals: If not consuming within a few days, freeze meals in individual portions. Use freezer-safe containers and remove excess air to prevent freezer burn.

7. Thawing Safely: Thaw frozen meals in the refrigerator or use the microwave's defrost setting. In order to stop bacteria from growing, do not leave them at room temperature.

8. Reheating Guidelines: Reheat meals to an internal temperature of 165°F (74°C) to ensure they are safe to eat. Use a food thermometer for accuracy.

9. Keep a Clean Fridge: Regularly clean and sanitize your refrigerator to prevent the growth of harmful bacteria.

10. Check for Signs of Spoilage: Periodically check the color, texture, and odor of stored items. Discard anything showing signs of spoilage to ensure food safety.

By following these guidelines, you can maintain the quality and safety of both your ingredients and prepared meals, ensuring a positive and healthy meal prep experience.

CHAPTER 4

STAPLE MEAL PREP COMPONENTS

Staple meal prep components are the essential ingredients that form the foundation of balanced and versatile meals. Incorporating these components into your meal prep routine ensures that you have a variety of options to create nutritious and satisfying dishes.

Here are some staple meal prep components to consider:

1. Proteins
Examples: Chicken breasts, lean ground turkey, tofu, tempeh, beans, lentils, and eggs.
Purpose: Proteins are crucial for muscle repair and overall body function. Prepare proteins in various ways to add diversity to your meals.

2. Whole Grains
Examples: Brown rice, quinoa, whole wheat pasta, barley, and oats.
Purpose: Whole grains provide complex carbohydrates and fiber, offering sustained energy and supporting digestive health.

3. Vegetables
Examples: Broccoli, spinach, bell peppers, carrots, zucchini, and cauliflower.
Purpose: Packed with vitamins, minerals, and fiber, vegetables add color, flavor, and nutritional value to your meals.

4. Healthy Fats
Examples: Avocado, olive oil, nuts, seeds, and fatty fish (salmon, tuna).
Purpose: Healthy fats are essential for heart health, satiety, and absorption of fat-soluble vitamins.

5. Leafy Greens
Examples: Kale, spinach, arugula, and Swiss chard.
Purpose: Leafy greens are nutrient-dense and versatile, suitable for salads, wraps, or sautés.

6. Fresh Herbs
Examples: Basil, cilantro, parsley, and mint.
Purpose: Herbs enhance the flavor of dishes without added calories or sodium, contributing to a vibrant and aromatic meal.

7. Low-Fat Dairy or Dairy Alternatives
Examples: Greek yogurt, low-fat cheese, or plant-based alternatives.

Purpose: Dairy provides calcium and protein, essential for bone health and overall nutrition.

8. Berries

Examples: Blueberries, strawberries, raspberries, and blackberries.

Purpose: Berries are rich in antioxidants, vitamins, and fiber, making them a nutritious addition to breakfasts or snacks.

9. Lean Cuts of Meat

Examples: Turkey, chicken, pork loin, and lean cuts of beef.

Purpose: Lean meats provide high-quality protein without excessive saturated fats, supporting muscle health.

10. Whole-Grain Bread or Wraps

Examples:Whole-grain bread, tortillas, or wraps.

Purpose: Use these as a base for sandwiches, wraps, or quick and easy meals.

11. Canned Beans

Examples: Chickpeas, black beans, kidney beans, and lentils.

Purpose: Canned beans are a convenient source of plant-based protein and fiber, perfect for salads, soups, or wraps.

12. Canned Tomatoes

Examples: Diced tomatoes, crushed tomatoes, or tomato sauce.

Purpose: Canned tomatoes serve as a versatile base for sauces, soups, stews, and casseroles.

13. Spices and Seasonings

Examples:.Garlic powder, cumin, paprika, and Italian seasoning.

Purpose: Spices add depth and flavor to your meals without added calories or sodium.

14. Broth or Stock

Examples: Vegetable broth, chicken broth, or beef broth.

Purpose: Broth enhances the flavor of soups, stews, and rice dishes, providing a savory base.

15. Hummus

Purpose: Hummus serves as a flavorful and nutritious dip or spread, complementing veggies, sandwiches, or wraps.

16. Nut Butter

Examples: Peanut butter, almond butter, or sunflower seed butter.

Purpose: Nut butters are rich in healthy fats and protein, making them a versatile addition to snacks or breakfast.

17. Grilled or Roasted Vegetables
Examples: Asparagus, eggplant, bell peppers, and cherry tomatoes.
Purpose: Preparing grilled or roasted vegetables in advance adds a delicious side to meals or a topping for salads.

18. Hard-Boiled Eggs
Purpose:.Hard-boiled eggs are a convenient and protein-rich snack or topping for salads.

19. Prepared Salad Greens
Examples: Mixed greens, arugula, or spinach.
Purpose: Having pre-washed and prepped salad greens on hand streamlines the process of creating quick and healthy salads.
20. Prepared Salad Dressings
Examples: Olive oil and balsamic vinegar, vinaigrettes, or yogurt-based dressings.
Purpose: Keep a variety of dressings to add flavor to salads without excessive added sugars or unhealthy fats.

By incorporating these staple components into your meal prep routine, you can create a diverse range of delicious and nutritionally balanced meals while saving time and promoting healthy eating habits.

CHAPTER 5

MEAL PREPS AND RECIPES (50 HEART-HEALTHY RECIPES)

Below are fifty heart-healthy recipes with nutritional components for each serving, along with a bonus heart-healthy smoothie recipe. These recipes aim to cater to various taste preferences while providing easy-to-follow instructions:

1. GRILLED LEMON HERB CHICKEN WITH QUINOA SALAD

Ingredients:
- 4 boneless, skinless chicken breasts
- 1 lemon (juiced and zested)
- 2 cloves garlic (minced)
- 1 teaspoon dried oregano
- 1 teaspoon dried thyme
- Salt and pepper to taste
- 1 cup quinoa (cooked)
- Cherry tomatoes, cucumber, and red onion for the salad
- Fresh parsley (chopped)

Nutritional Components (per serving):
- Protein: 25g
- Fiber: 6g

- Healthy Fats: 4g
- Vitamin C: 30% of daily value

Instructions:
- In a bowl, mix lemon juice, zest, minced garlic, oregano, thyme, salt, and pepper.
- Marinate chicken in the mixture for at least 30 minutes.
- Grill chicken until cooked through.
- Prepare a salad with cooked quinoa, cherry tomatoes, cucumber, and red onion.
- Serve grilled chicken on top of the quinoa salad, garnished with fresh parsley.

2. BAKED SALMON WITH ROASTED VEGETABLES

Ingredients:
- 4 salmon filets
- 1 tablespoon olive oil
- 1 teaspoon Dijon mustard
- 1 teaspoon honey
- 1 teaspoon dried dill
- Salt and pepper to taste
- Mixed vegetables (e.g., broccoli, bell peppers, and carrots)

Nutritional Components (per serving):
- Omega-3 Fatty Acids: 2.5g
- Fiber: 4g
- Vitamin A: 120% of daily value
- Vitamin D: 30% of daily value

Instructions:
- Preheat the oven to 400°F (200°C).
- In a small bowl, mix olive oil, Dijon mustard, honey, dried dill, salt, and pepper.
- Place salmon filets on a baking sheet, brush with the mixture, and bake for 15-20 minutes.
- Toss mixed vegetables in the remaining mixture and roast until tender.
- Serve baked salmon over a bed of roasted vegetables.

3. QUINOA AND BLACK BEAN STUFFED PEPPERS

Ingredients:
- 4 large bell peppers (halved and seeds removed)
- 1 cup quinoa (cooked)
- 1 can black beans (drained and rinsed)
- 1 cup corn kernels
- 1 cup cherry tomatoes (halved)
- 1 teaspoon cumin

- 1 teaspoon chili powder
- 1/2 teaspoon smoked paprika
- Salt and pepper to taste
- 1 cup shredded low-fat cheese (optional)

Nutritional Components (per serving):
- Protein: 15g
- Fiber: 9g
- Vitamin C: 160% of daily value
- Iron: 15% of daily value

Instructions:
- Preheat the oven to 375°F (190°C).
- In a bowl, mix cooked quinoa, black beans, corn, cherry tomatoes, cumin, chili powder, smoked paprika, salt, and pepper.
- Stuff each bell pepper half with the quinoa and black bean mixture.
- If desired, sprinkle shredded cheese on top.
- Bake for 25-30 minutes or until the peppers are tender.

4. MEDITERRANEAN CHICKPEA SALAD

Ingredients:
- 1 can chickpeas (drained and rinsed)
- Cucumber, tomatoes, red onion, and bell peppers (chopped)
- Feta cheese (crumbled)

- Kalamata olives (sliced)
- Olive oil, lemon juice, oregano, salt, and pepper for dressing.

Nutritional Components (per serving):
- Protein: 10g
- Fiber: 8g
- Healthy Fats: 6g
- Vitamin K: 60% of daily value

Instructions:
- Mix chickpeas, vegetables, and feta in a bowl.
- Whisk together olive oil, lemon juice, oregano, salt, and pepper for the dressing.
- Toss salad with dressing until well combined.

5. VEGETARIAN LENTIL SOUP

Ingredients:
- 1 cup dry lentils (rinsed)
- Carrots, celery, onion, and garlic (chopped)
- Vegetable broth
- Crushed tomatoes
- Cumin, coriander, smoked paprika, salt, and pepper.

Nutritional Components (per serving):
- Protein: 18g
- Fiber: 12g
- Iron: 25% of daily value
- Folate: 90% of daily value

Instructions:
- Combine lentils, vegetables, broth, and tomatoes in a pot.
- Add spices and simmer until lentils are tender.
- Adjust seasoning and serve.

6. SHRIMP AND VEGETABLE STIR-FRY

Ingredients:
- Shrimp (peeled and deveined)
- Broccoli, bell peppers, snap peas, and carrots (sliced)
- Ginger and garlic (minced)
- Low-sodium soy sauce, sesame oil, and honey.

Nutritional Components (per serving):
- Protein: 20g
- Fiber: 4g
- Omega-3 Fatty Acids: 300mg
- Vitamin C: 80% of daily value

Instructions:
- Stir-fry shrimp and vegetables in sesame oil.
- Add ginger and garlic, then pour in soy sauce and honey.
- Cook until shrimp are pink and vegetables are crisp-tender.

7. SWEET POTATO AND BLACK BEAN ENCHILADAS

Ingredients:
- Sweet potatoes (cooked and mashed)
- Black beans (canned, drained, and rinsed)
- Whole-grain tortillas
- Enchilada sauce, cumin, chili powder, and shredded cheese.

Nutritional Components (per serving):
- Protein: 15g
- Fiber: 8g
- Vitamin A: 120% of daily value
- Calcium: 20% of daily value

Instructions:
- Mix sweet potatoes and black beans.
- Fill tortillas with the mixture, roll, and place in a baking dish.
- Top with enchilada sauce and cheese, then bake until bubbly.

8. OVEN-BAKED HERB-CRUSTED COD

Ingredients:
- Cod filets
- Whole wheat breadcrumbs, parsley, thyme, lemon zest, and garlic (combined)
- Olive oil, salt, and pepper.

Nutritional Components (per serving):
- Protein: 22g
- Omega-3 Fatty Acids: 500mg
- Vitamin D: 50% of daily value
- Vitamin B12: 60% of daily value

Instructions:
- Coat cod filets in olive oil and the herb mixture.
- Bake until the fish is cooked through and flakes easily.

9. ASIAN-INSPIRED QUINOA BOWL

Ingredients:
- Quinoa (cooked)
- Edamame, shredded carrots, red cabbage, and scallions
- Sesame oil, soy sauce, ginger, and rice vinegar for dressing.

Nutritional Components (per serving):
- Protein: 12g
- Fiber: 8g
- Vitamin K: 40% of daily value
- Iron: 15% of daily value

Instructions:
- Assemble quinoa and vegetables in a bowl.
- Whisk together sesame oil, soy sauce, ginger, and rice vinegar for the dressing.
- Drizzle the dressing over the bowl and toss.

10. CAULIFLOWER AND CHICKPEA CURRY

Ingredients:
- Cauliflower florets
- Chickpeas (canned, drained, and rinsed)
- Onion, garlic, and ginger (minced)
- Curry powder, cumin, turmeric, and coconut milk.

Nutritional Components (per serving):
- Protein: 14g
- Fiber: 10g
- Vitamin C: 80% of daily value
- Magnesium: 15% of daily value

Instructions:

- Sauté onion, garlic, and ginger in a pot.
- Add cauliflower, chickpeas, and spices, then pour in coconut milk.
- Simmer until the cauliflower is tender.

11. MANGO AVOCADO QUINOA SALAD

Ingredients:

- Quinoa (cooked)
- Ripe mango (diced)
- Avocado (sliced)
- Red onion, cucumber, and bell pepper (chopped)
- Fresh cilantro
- Lime juice, olive oil, salt, and pepper for dressing.

Nutritional Components (per serving):

- Fiber: 7g
- Healthy Fats: 10g
- Vitamin C: 50% of daily value
- Vitamin E: 15% of daily value

Instructions:

- Combine quinoa, mango, avocado, vegetables, and cilantro in a bowl.
- Whisk together lime juice, olive oil, salt, and pepper for the dressing.

- Toss the salad with the dressing until well coated.

12. TUSCAN WHITE BEAN AND SPINACH SOUP

Ingredients:
- Cannellini beans (canned, drained, and rinsed)
- Spinach leaves
- Garlic, onion, and carrots (chopped)
- Vegetable broth
- Italian seasoning, rosemary, salt, and pepper.

Nutritional Components (per serving):
- Protein: 10g
- Fiber: 8g
- Vitamin A: 120% of daily value
- Vitamin K: 90% of daily value

Instructions:
- Sauté garlic, onion, and carrots in a pot.
- Add beans, spinach, broth, and spices. Simmer until vegetables are tender.

13. TURKEY AND VEGETABLE STUFFED BELL PEPPERS

Ingredients:
- Lean ground turkey
- Bell peppers (halved and seeds removed)
- Quinoa (cooked)
- Zucchini, tomatoes, and corn (chopped)
- Taco seasoning, cumin, and salsa.

Nutritional Components (per serving):
- Protein: 20g
- Fiber: 6g
- Vitamin C: 150% of daily value
- Selenium: 45% of daily value

Instructions:
- Brown turkey in a skillet, then mix with quinoa, vegetables, and spices.
- Stuff bell peppers with the mixture and bake until peppers are tender.

14. PESTO ZOODLES WITH CHERRY TOMATOES
- Ingredients:
- Zucchini (spiralized into noodles)
- Cherry tomatoes (halved)
- Pesto sauce (homemade or store-bought)
- Pine nuts (toasted)

- Parmesan cheese (grated)

Nutritional Components (per serving):
- Fiber: 4g
- Healthy Fats: 15g
- Vitamin A: 25% of daily value
- Vitamin C: 40% of daily value

Instructions:
- Sauté zoodles until tender.
- Toss zoodles with pesto sauce, cherry tomatoes, and top with toasted pine nuts and Parmesan.

15. SALMON AND ASPARAGUS FOIL PACKETS

Ingredients:
- Salmon filets
- Asparagus spears
- Lemon slices
- Garlic (minced)
- Dill, salt, and pepper.

Nutritional Components (per serving):
- Protein: 25g
- Omega-3 Fatty Acids: 1g
- Vitamin C: 30% of daily value
- Vitamin D: 25% of daily value

Instructions:

- Place salmon, asparagus, and lemon slices on a sheet of foil.
- Sprinkle it with minced garlic, dill, salt, and pepper. Seal the packets and bake until the salmon is cooked.

16. CHICKPEA AND VEGETABLE STIR-FRY

Ingredients:

- Chickpeas (canned, drained, and rinsed)
- Broccoli, bell peppers, snap peas, and carrots (sliced)
- Ginger and garlic (minced)
- Low-sodium soy sauce, sesame oil, and honey.

Nutritional Components (per serving):

- Protein: 15g
- Fiber: 8g
- Vitamin C: 70% of daily value
- Iron: 20% of daily value

Instructions:

- Stir-fry chickpeas and vegetables in sesame oil.
- Add ginger and garlic, then pour in soy sauce and honey.

- Cook until vegetables are crisp-tender.

17. CAPRESE QUINOA SALAD

Ingredients:
- Quinoa (cooked)
- Cherry tomatoes (halved)
- Fresh mozzarella balls (mini)
- Fresh basil leaves
- Balsamic glaze
- Olive oil, salt, and pepper.

Nutritional Components (per serving):
- Protein: 10g
- Healthy Fats: 8g
- Vitamin A: 15% of daily value
- Calcium: 15% of daily value

Instructions:
- Combine quinoa, tomatoes, mozzarella, and basil in a bowl.
- Drizzle with olive oil and balsamic glaze, season with salt and pepper, and toss.

18. LEMON GARLIC SHRIMP WITH BROCCOLI

Ingredients:
- Shrimp (peeled and deveined)
- Broccoli florets

- Lemon juice and zest
- Garlic (minced)
- Olive oil, salt, and pepper.

Nutritional Components (per serving):
- Protein: 20g
- Fiber: 5g
- Vitamin C: 90% of daily value
- Vitamin K: 100% of daily value

Instructions:
- Sauté shrimp in olive oil with minced garlic until pink.
- Add broccoli, lemon juice, and zest. Cook until broccoli is tender.

19. MUSHROOM AND SPINACH STUFFED CHICKEN BREAST

Ingredients:
- Chicken breasts
- Mushrooms (sliced)
- Spinach leaves
- Garlic (minced)
- Low-fat cream cheese
- Thyme, salt, and pepper.

Nutritional Components (per serving):
- Protein: 30g
- Fiber: 3g
- Vitamin D: 15% of daily value
- Calcium: 8% of daily value

Instructions:
- Sauté mushrooms and garlic, then mix with spinach and cream cheese.
- Cut a pocket in each chicken breast, stuff with the mixture, and bake until cooked.

20. PEACH AND WALNUT QUINOA BOWL

Ingredients:
- Quinoa (cooked)
- Fresh peaches (sliced)
- Walnuts (chopped)
- Greek yogurt
- Honey
- Cinnamon.

Nutritional Components (per serving):
- Protein: 8g
- Healthy Fats: 10g
- Vitamin C: 15% of daily value
- Iron: 10% of daily value

Instructions:
- Combine quinoa, peaches, and walnuts in a bowl.
- Top with a dollop of Greek yogurt, drizzle with honey, and sprinkle with cinnamon.

21. CABBAGE AND LENTIL STEW

Ingredients:
- Green or red cabbage (shredded)
- Lentils (rinsed and drained)
- Tomatoes (diced)
- Onion, garlic, and carrots (chopped)
- Vegetable broth
- Cumin, coriander, turmeric, and bay leaves.

Nutritional Components (per serving):
- Protein: 15g
- Fiber: 12g
- Vitamin A: 80% of daily value
- Iron: 25% of daily value

Instructions:
- Sauté onions, garlic, and carrots until softened.
- Add cabbage, lentils, tomatoes, broth, and spices. Simmer until lentils are tender.

22. CILANTRO LIME CHICKEN WITH AVOCADO SALSA

Ingredients:
- Chicken breasts
- Fresh cilantro (chopped)
- Lime juice and zest
- Avocado, tomatoes, red onion, and jalapeño for salsa.
- Olive oil, cumin, and garlic powder.

Nutritional Components (per serving):
- Protein: 25g
- Healthy Fats: 10g
- Vitamin C: 40% of daily value
- Vitamin K: 30% of daily value

Instructions:
- Mix cilantro, lime juice, lime zest, cumin, garlic powder, and olive oil.
- Marinate chicken and grill until fully cooked. Top with avocado salsa.

23. MUSHROOM BARLEY RISOTTO

Ingredients:
- Pearl barley (cooked)
- Mushrooms (sliced)
- Onion and garlic (chopped)

- Low-sodium vegetable broth
- Parmesan cheese (grated)
- Thyme, salt, and pepper.

Nutritional Components (per serving):
- Protein: 10g
- Fiber: 8g
- Vitamin D: 10% of daily value
- Calcium: 15% of daily value

Instructions:
- Sauté mushrooms, onions, and garlic until tender.
- Add cooked barley, thyme, broth, and simmer until the liquid is absorbed.
- Stir in Parmesan cheese and season with salt and pepper.

24. STUFFED ACORN SQUASH WITH QUINOA AND CRANBERRIES

Ingredients:
- Acorn squash (halved and seeds removed)
- Quinoa (cooked)
- Dried cranberries
- Pecans (chopped)
- Maple syrup
- Cinnamon, nutmeg, and salt.

Nutritional Components (per serving):

- Protein: 8g
- Fiber: 7g
- Vitamin A: 180% of daily value
- Iron: 10% of daily value

Instructions:

- Roast acorn squash until tender.
- Mix quinoa, cranberries, pecans, maple syrup, cinnamon, nutmeg, and salt.
- Fill the squash halves with the quinoa mixture.

25. PESTO SALMON WITH ROASTED VEGETABLES

Ingredients:

- Salmon filets
- Zucchini, cherry tomatoes, and red onion (sliced)
- Pesto sauce (homemade or store-bought)
- Olive oil, salt, and pepper.

Nutritional Components (per serving):

- Protein: 20g
- Omega-3 Fatty Acids: 1.5g
- Vitamin C: 60% of daily value
- Vitamin K: 80% of daily value

Instructions:

- Preheat the oven to 400°F (200°C).
- Place salmon and vegetables on a baking sheet, drizzle with olive oil, and season with salt and pepper.
- Bake until salmon is cooked through and vegetables are tender.

26. VEGETARIAN STUFFED BELL PEPPERS WITH QUINOA AND BLACK BEANS

Ingredients:

- Bell peppers (halved and seeds removed)
- Quinoa (cooked)
- Black beans (canned, drained, and rinsed)
- Corn, tomatoes, and green onions (chopped)
- Taco seasoning, cumin, and cilantro.

Nutritional Components (per serving):

- Protein: 12g
- Fiber: 7g
- Vitamin C: 120% of daily value
- Folate: 25% of daily value

Instructions:

- Mix quinoa, black beans, corn, tomatoes, green onions, taco seasoning, cumin, and cilantro.

- Stuff bell peppers with the mixture and bake until peppers are tender.

27. LEMON HERB TOFU STIR-FRY

Ingredients:
- Extra-firm tofu (pressed and cubed)
- Broccoli, bell peppers, snap peas, and carrots (sliced)
- Lemon juice and zest
- Garlic (minced)
- Soy sauce, ginger, and sesame oil.

Nutritional Components (per serving):
- Protein: 15g
- Fiber: 6g
- Vitamin C: 90% of daily value
- Iron: 20% of daily value

Instructions:
- Sauté tofu in sesame oil until golden.
- Add vegetables, garlic, soy sauce, ginger, lemon juice, and zest. Cook until vegetables are crisp-tender.

28. GREEK CHICKPEA SALAD

Ingredients:
- Chickpeas (canned, drained, and rinsed)
- Cucumber, cherry tomatoes, red onion, and Kalamata olives (chopped)
- Feta cheese (crumbled)
- Olive oil, lemon juice, oregano, salt, and pepper.

Nutritional Components (per serving):
- Protein: 10g
- Fiber: 8g
- Healthy Fats: 6g
- Vitamin K: 40% of daily value

Instructions:
- Combine chickpeas, vegetables, feta, and olives in a bowl.
- Whisk together olive oil, lemon juice, oregano, salt, and pepper for the dressing.
- Toss the salad with the dressing until well combined.

29. SPAGHETTI SQUASH WITH TOMATO BASIL SAUCE

Ingredients:
- Spaghetti squash (cooked and shredded)
- Tomatoes, garlic, and fresh basil (chopped)

- Olive oil, onion, red pepper flakes, salt, and pepper.

Nutritional Components (per serving):
- Fiber: 6g
- Vitamin C: 30% of daily value
- Vitamin K: 20% of daily value
- Manganese: 20% of daily value

Instructions:
- Sauté garlic and onion in olive oil until softened.
- Add tomatoes, fresh basil, red pepper flakes, salt, and pepper. Simmer until the sauce thickens.
- Serve over cooked and shredded spaghetti squash.

30. BLACKENED TILAPIA TACOS WITH CABBAGE SLAW

Ingredients:
- Tilapia filets
- Corn tortillas
- Cabbage, carrots, and cilantro (shredded)
- Lime juice and zest
- Blackening seasoning, cumin, and Greek yogurt.

Nutritional Components (per serving):
- Protein: 18g
- Fiber: 5g
- Vitamin C: 60% of daily value
- Calcium: 15% of daily value

Instructions:
- Coat tilapia with blackening seasoning and grill until cooked.
- Mix cabbage, carrots, cilantro, lime juice, and zest for the slaw.
- Assemble tacos with tilapia and slaw, and top with a dollop of Greek yogurt.

31. BAKED EGGPLANT PARMESAN

Ingredients:
- Eggplant slices
- Whole wheat breadcrumbs, Parmesan cheese, and fresh basil (combined)
- Marinara sauce (low sodium)
- Mozzarella cheese (part-skim)

Nutritional Components (per serving):
- Protein: 12g
- Fiber: 8g
- Vitamin A: 25% of daily value
- Calcium: 20% of daily value

Instructions:

- Dip eggplant slices in marinara, then coat with breadcrumb mixture.
- Layer in a baking dish with marinara and mozzarella. Bake until bubbly.

32. QUINOA AND VEGETABLE STUFFED PORTOBELLO MUSHROOMS

Ingredients:

- Portobello mushrooms (stems removed)
- Quinoa (cooked)
- Spinach, cherry tomatoes, and red bell pepper (chopped)
- Feta cheese (crumbled)
- Balsamic glaze

Nutritional Components (per serving):

- Protein: 10g
- Fiber: 6g
- Vitamin D: 15% of daily value
- Iron: 10% of daily value

Instructions:

- Roast portobello mushrooms until tender.
- Mix quinoa, vegetables, and feta. Stuff mushrooms and drizzle with balsamic glaze.

33. TERIYAKI TOFU AND VEGETABLE SKEWERS

Ingredients:
- Extra-firm tofu (cubed)
- Bell peppers, zucchini, and red onion (sliced)
- Teriyaki marinade (low sodium)
- Sesame seeds

Nutritional Components (per serving):
- Protein: 15g
- Fiber: 5g
- Vitamin C: 80% of daily value
- Iron: 15% of daily value

Instructions:
- Marinate tofu and vegetables in teriyaki sauce.
- Skewer and grill until tofu is golden and vegetables are charred. Sprinkle with sesame seeds.

34. WILD RICE AND CRANBERRY STUFFED ACORN SQUASH

Ingredients:
- Acorn squash (halved and seeds removed)
- Wild rice (cooked)

- Dried cranberries
- Pecans (chopped)
- Maple syrup
- Cinnamon and nutmeg

Nutritional Components (per serving):
- Protein: 8g
- Fiber: 7g
- Vitamin A: 160% of daily value
- Iron: 8% of daily value

Instructions:
- Roast acorn squash until tender.
- Mix wild rice, cranberries, pecans, maple syrup, cinnamon, and nutmeg. Fill the squash halves.

35. MANGO AVOCADO BLACK BEAN SALAD

Ingredients:
- Black beans (canned, drained, and rinsed)
- Mango and avocado (diced)
- Red onion, cilantro, and jalapeño (chopped)
- Lime juice
- Salt and pepper

Nutritional Components (per serving):
- Protein: 8g
- Fiber: 10g
- Vitamin C: 45% of daily value

- Healthy Fats: 10g

Instructions:
- Combine black beans, mango, avocado, red onion, cilantro, and jalapeño.
- Squeeze lime juice over the salad and season with salt and pepper.

36. WHOLE GRAIN PENNE WITH ROASTED VEGETABLES AND PESTO

Ingredients:
- Whole grain penne pasta (cooked)
- Broccoli, cherry tomatoes, and bell peppers (roasted)
- Pesto sauce (homemade or store-bought)
- Parmesan cheese (grated)

Nutritional Components (per serving):
- Protein: 12g
- Fiber: 6g
- Vitamin A: 20% of daily value
- Calcium: 10% of daily value

Instructions:
- Toss roasted vegetables with cooked whole grain penne.
- Mix in pesto sauce and top with grated Parmesan.

37. CHIA SEED PUDDING WITH MIXED BERRIES

Ingredients:
- Chia seeds
- Almond milk
- Mixed berries (strawberries, blueberries, raspberries)
- Honey or maple syrup

Nutritional Components (per serving):
- Protein: 5g
- Fiber: 10g
- Antioxidants: High
- Omega-3 Fatty Acids: 2g

Instructions:
- Mix chia seeds with almond milk and refrigerate overnight.
- Top with mixed berries and drizzle with honey or maple syrup.

38. BRUSSELS SPROUTS AND SWEET POTATO HASH

Ingredients:
- Brussels sprouts (shredded)
- Sweet potatoes (grated)

- Onion and garlic (chopped)
- Olive oil
- Paprika, cumin, and thyme

Nutritional Components (per serving):
- Protein: 5g
- Fiber: 8g
- Vitamin A: 160% of daily value
- Vitamin C: 80% of daily value

Instructions:
- Sauté onions and garlic in olive oil until softened.
- Add shredded Brussels sprouts, grated sweet potatoes, paprika, cumin, and thyme. Cook until golden.

39. PINEAPPLE CHICKEN LETTUCE WRAPS

Ingredients:
- Chicken breasts (cooked and shredded)
- Pineapple (diced)
- Red bell pepper, cucumber, and carrots (julienned)
- Bibb lettuce leaves
- Hoisin sauce and soy sauce

Nutritional Components (per serving):
- Protein: 15g

- Fiber: 4g
- Vitamin C: 70% of daily value
- Vitamin A: 120% of daily value

Instructions:
- Mix shredded chicken with pineapple, bell pepper, cucumber, and carrots.
- Drizzle with a mixture of hoisin sauce and soy sauce. Serve in lettuce wraps.

40. EGG WHITE OMELET WITH SPINACH AND FETA

Ingredients:
- Egg whites
- Fresh spinach leaves
- Feta cheese (crumbled)
- Cherry tomatoes (sliced)
- Olive oil
- Salt and pepper

Nutritional Components (per serving):
- Protein: 15g
- Vitamin A: 25% of daily value
- Calcium: 15% of daily value
- Healthy Fats: 6g

Instructions:

- Whisk egg whites and pour into a heated pan with olive oil.
- Add spinach, feta, and tomatoes. Cook until eggs are set. Season with salt and pepper.

41. CAULIFLOWER RICE STIR-FRY WITH TOFU

Ingredients:

- Cauliflower rice (store-bought or homemade)
- Extra-firm tofu (cubed)
- Mixed vegetables (broccoli, carrots, peas)
- Low-sodium soy sauce
- Ginger and garlic (minced)
- Sesame oil

Nutritional Components (per serving):

- Protein: 12g
- Fiber: 8g
- Vitamin C: 60% of daily value
- Iron: 15% of daily value

Instructions:

- Sauté tofu in sesame oil until golden.
- Add cauliflower rice, mixed vegetables, ginger, garlic, and soy sauce. Stir-fry until vegetables are tender.

42. SWEET POTATO AND CHICKPEA CURRY

Ingredients:
- Sweet potatoes (cubed)
- Chickpeas (canned, drained, and rinsed)
- Coconut milk (light)
- Curry powder, cumin, and coriander
- Spinach leaves
- Lime juice

Nutritional Components (per serving):
- Protein: 10g
- Fiber: 8g
- Vitamin A: 300% of daily value
- Iron: 20% of daily value

Instructions:
- Simmer sweet potatoes, chickpeas, coconut milk, and spices until sweet potatoes are tender.
- Stir in spinach and lime juice before serving.

43. TURKEY AND VEGETABLE QUINOA BOWL

Ingredients:
- Ground turkey
- Quinoa (cooked)
- Bell peppers, zucchini, and cherry tomatoes (chopped)
- Olive oil
- Italian seasoning, garlic powder, salt, and pepper

Nutritional Components (per serving):
- Protein: 20g
- Fiber: 6g
- Vitamin C: 80% of daily value
- Healthy Fats: 8g

Instructions:
- Brown ground turkey in olive oil with Italian seasoning and garlic powder.
- Mix in chopped vegetables and cook until tender. Serve over quinoa.

44. BLUEBERRY ALMOND OVERNIGHT OATS
Ingredients:
- Rolled oats
- Almond milk
- Blueberries

- Almonds (sliced)
- Chia seeds
- Vanilla extract

Nutritional Components (per serving):
- Protein: 10g
- Fiber: 8g
- Antioxidants: High
- Healthy Fats: 12g

Instructions:
- Combine oats, almond milk, blueberries, almonds, chia seeds, and vanilla extract in a jar.
- Refrigerate overnight and enjoy a quick and nutritious breakfast.

45. SESAME GINGER SALMON BOWL

Ingredients:
- Salmon filets
- Brown rice (cooked)
- Broccoli florets
- Carrots (julienned)
- Sesame oil
- Ginger and garlic (minced)
- Low-sodium soy sauce

Nutritional Components (per serving):
- Protein: 25g
- Omega-3 Fatty Acids: 1.5g
- Vitamin C: 50% of daily value
- Iron: 15% of daily value

Instructions:
- Roast salmon, broccoli, and carrots in sesame oil, ginger, garlic, and soy sauce.
- Serve over cooked brown rice.

46. ZUCCHINI NOODLES WITH PESTO AND CHERRY TOMATOES

Ingredients:
- Zucchini (spiralized into noodles)
- Pesto sauce (homemade or store-bought)
- Cherry tomatoes (halved)
- Pine nuts (toasted)
- Parmesan cheese (grated)

Nutritional Components (per serving):
- Protein: 8g
- Fiber: 4g
- Vitamin A: 15% of daily value
- Calcium: 10% of daily value

Instructions:
- Sauté zucchini noodles until tender.
- Toss with pesto sauce, cherry tomatoes, toasted pine nuts, and Parmesan.

47. MEDITERRANEAN CHICKPEA SALAD

Ingredients:
- Chickpeas (canned, drained, and rinsed)
- Cucumber, cherry tomatoes, red onion, and Kalamata olives (chopped)
- Feta cheese (crumbled)
- Olive oil, lemon juice, oregano, salt, and pepper

Nutritional Components (per serving):
- Protein: 12g
- Fiber: 8g
- Healthy Fats: 10g
- Vitamin C: 30% of daily value

Instructions:
- Combine chickpeas, vegetables, feta, and olives in a bowl.
- Whisk together olive oil, lemon juice, oregano, salt, and pepper for the dressing.
- Toss the salad with the dressing until well combined.

48. CRISPY BAKED COD WITH QUINOA PILAF

Ingredients:
- Cod filets
- Quinoa (cooked)
- Spinach, bell peppers, and cherry tomatoes (chopped)
- Lemon juice and zest
- Olive oil
- Paprika, thyme, salt, and pepper

Nutritional Components (per serving):
- Protein: 20g
- Fiber: 6g
- Vitamin C: 45% of daily value
- Omega-3 Fatty Acids: 0.8g

Instructions:
- Season cod with paprika, thyme, salt, and pepper. Bake until crispy.
- Mix quinoa with spinach, bell peppers, cherry tomatoes, lemon juice, and zest.

49. PUMPKIN AND LENTIL SOUP
Ingredients:
- Red lentils (rinsed and drained)
- Pumpkin puree

- Carrots, celery, and onion (chopped)
- Vegetable broth
- Cumin, coriander, and nutmeg
- Greek yogurt (optional for topping)

Nutritional Components (per serving):
- Protein: 15g
- Fiber: 10g
- Vitamin A: 200% of daily value
- Iron: 25% of daily value

Instructions:
- Sauté carrots, celery, and onion until softened.
- Add lentils, pumpkin puree, broth, cumin, coriander, and nutmeg. Simmer until lentils are tender.

50. TURKEY AND BLACK BEAN STUFFED PEPPERS

Ingredients:
- Ground turkey
- Black beans (canned, drained, and rinsed)
- Quinoa (cooked)
- Bell peppers (halved)
- Tomato sauce
- Cumin, chili powder, and garlic powder

Nutritional Components (per serving):
- Protein: 18g
- Fiber: 8g
- Vitamin C: 160% of daily value
- Folate: 20% of daily value

Instructions:
- Brown ground turkey with cumin, chili powder, and garlic powder.
- Mix with black beans and quinoa. Stuff into halved bell peppers and bake until peppers are tender.

HEART-HEALTHY SMOOTHIE: BERRY BLAST:

Ingredients:
- 1 cup mixed berries (blueberries, strawberries, raspberries)
- 1/2 banana
- 1 cup low-fat Greek yogurt
- 1 tablespoon chia seeds
- 1/2 cup almond milk
- Ice cubes (optional)

Nutritional Components (per serving):
- Antioxidants: High
- Probiotics: Present in Greek yogurt
- Fiber: 8g
- Vitamin C: 80% of daily value

Instructions:

- Blend mixed berries, banana, Greek yogurt, chia seeds, and almond milk until smooth.
- Add ice cubes if a colder consistency is desired.
- Pour into a glass and enjoy this refreshing and heart-healthy smoothie.

Feel free to customize these recipes based on individual taste preferences and dietary needs. These dishes offer a combination of lean proteins, whole grains, vegetables, and heart-healthy fats to support cardiovascular health. Enjoy your delicious and nutritious meals.

CHAPTER 6

SIX WEEKLY MEAL PLANS

WEEK 1 - JUMPSTART YOUR WELLNESS: A FRESH WEEK OF DASH DELIGHTS

Here's a diverse and flavorful weekly meal plan for you. Please keep in mind that the serving sizes and nutritional values are approximate and may vary based on specific ingredients and preparation methods.

Day 1: Energizing Start

Breakfast: Berry Almond Smoothie Bowl

Ingredients:
- 1 cup mixed berries (strawberries, blueberries, raspberries)
- 1 banana
- 1/2 cup almond milk
- 1/4 cup almonds (sliced)
- 2 tablespoons chia seeds
- Granola for topping

Nutritional Components (per serving):
- Protein: 10g
- Fiber: 12g
- Healthy Fats: 15g
- Vitamin C: 40% of daily value

Instructions:
- Blend mixed berries, banana, and almond milk until smooth.
- Pour into a bowl and top with sliced almonds, chia seeds, and granola.

Lunch: Quinoa and Chickpea Salad Bowl

Ingredients:
- 1 cup quinoa (cooked)
- 1 cup chickpeas (canned, drained, and rinsed)
- 1 cup cucumber (diced)
- 1 cup cherry tomatoes (halved)
- 1/4 cup red onion (finely chopped)
- Feta cheese (optional)
- Olive oil and lemon juice for dressing

Nutritional Components (per serving):
- Protein: 15g
- Fiber: 8g
- Healthy Fats: 10g
- Vitamin C: 25% of daily value

Instructions:
- In a bowl, combine quinoa, chickpeas, cucumber, cherry tomatoes, and red onion.
- Drizzle with olive oil and lemon juice. Add feta cheese if desired.

Dinner: Grilled Chicken with Roasted Vegetables

Ingredients:
- 6 oz chicken breast
- 1 cup broccoli florets
- 1 cup carrots (sliced)
- 1 cup bell peppers (sliced)
- Olive oil, garlic, rosemary (for marinade)
- Salt and pepper to taste

Nutritional Components (per serving):
- Protein: 30g
- Fiber: 7g
- Healthy Fats: 8g
- Vitamin A: 150% of daily value

Instructions:
- Marinate chicken in olive oil, minced garlic, and rosemary. Grill until cooked.
- Toss broccoli, carrots, and bell peppers in olive oil, salt, and pepper. Roast until tender.

Snack: Greek Yogurt with Honey

Ingredients:
- 1 cup Greek yogurt
- 1 tablespoon honey

Nutritional Components (per serving):
- Protein: 20g
- Carbohydrates: 25g
- Healthy Fats: 5g

Instructions:
- Spoon Greek yogurt into a bowl.
- Drizzle with honey. Enjoy a simple and satisfying snack!

Dessert: Dark Chocolate-Dipped Strawberries

Ingredients:
- Fresh strawberries
- Dark chocolate (70% cocoa or higher)

Nutritional Components (per serving):
- Fiber: 3g
- Antioxidants: High
- Natural Sugars

Instructions:
- Melt dark chocolate.
- Dip each strawberry into the chocolate. Allow to cool and harden.

Grocery List for Day 1

Mixed berries, Banana, Almond milk, Almonds, Chia seeds, Granola, Quinoa, Chickpeas, Cucumber, Cherry tomatoes, Red onion, Feta cheese, Olive oil, Lemon, Chicken breast, Broccoli, Carrots, Bell peppers, Garlic, Rosemary, Greek yogurt, Honey, Fresh strawberries, Dark chocolate.

Day 2: Fresh Start

Breakfast: Avocado Toast with Poached Egg

Ingredients:
- 2 slices whole-grain bread
- 1 ripe avocado
- 2 eggs
- Salt and pepper to taste
- Red pepper flakes (optional)

Nutritional Components (per serving):
- Protein: 12g
- Fiber: 8g
- Healthy Fats: 20g
- Vitamin A: 15% of daily value

Instructions:

- Toast the whole-grain bread slices.
- Mash the ripe avocado and spread it on the toast.
- Poach the eggs and place them on top. Season with salt, pepper, and red pepper flakes if desired.

Lunch: Lentil and Vegetable Wrap

Ingredients:

- 1 cup cooked lentils
- Whole wheat wrap
- 1 cup mixed vegetables (bell peppers, spinach, tomatoes)
- Hummus for spreading

Nutritional Components (per serving):

- Protein: 15g
- Fiber: 10g
- Healthy Fats: 8g
- Iron: 20% of daily value

Instructions:

- In a whole wheat wrap, spread a layer of hummus.
- Fill it with cooked lentils and mixed vegetables.

- Roll it up and enjoy a satisfying and nutritious wrap.

Dinner: Baked Cod with Lemon and Herbs

Ingredients:
- 6 oz cod filet
- 1 lemon
- Fresh thyme
- Rosemary
- Olive oil
- Salt and pepper to taste

Nutritional Components (per serving):
- Protein: 30g
- Fiber: 2g
- Healthy Fats: 10g
- Vitamin C: 45% of daily value

Instructions:
- Preheat the oven to 375°F (190°C).
- Place the cod filet on a baking sheet.
- Season with olive oil, fresh thyme, rosemary, salt, and pepper.
- Bake for 15-20 minutes or until the cod is cooked through.

Snack: Sliced Apple with Almond Butter

Ingredients:
- 1 apple (sliced)
- 2 tablespoons almond butter

Nutritional Components (per serving):
- Protein: 4g
- Fiber: 6g
- Healthy Fats: 14g
- Carbohydrates: 20g

Instructions:
- Slice the apple into wedges.
- Dip in almond butter for a tasty and balanced snack.

Dessert: Mixed Berry Parfait

Ingredients:
- Mixed berries (strawberries, blueberries, raspberries)
- Greek yogurt
- Granola

Nutritional Components (per serving):
- Protein: 15g
- Fiber: 8g
- Healthy Fats: 6g

- Vitamin C: 30% of daily value

Instructions:
- In a glass, layer Greek yogurt with mixed berries and granola.

Grocery List for Day 2

Whole-grain bread, Avocado, Eggs, Red pepper flakes, Lentils, Whole wheat wrap, Mixed vegetables (bell peppers, spinach, tomatoes), Hummus, Cod filet, Lemon, Fresh thyme, Rosemary, Olive oil, Sliced apple, Almond butter, Greek yogurt, Granola.

Day 3: Plant-Powered Delight

Breakfast: Chia Seed Pudding with Mango

Ingredients:
- 3 tablespoons chia seeds
- 1 cup almond milk
- 1 ripe mango (diced)

Nutritional Components (per serving):
- Protein: 8g
- Fiber: 15g
- Healthy Fats: 10g
- Vitamin C: 60% of daily value

Instructions:
- Mix chia seeds with almond milk in a jar.
- Refrigerate overnight.
- In the morning, top with diced mango for a refreshing and fiber-rich breakfast.

Lunch: Mediterranean Chickpea Salad

Ingredients:
- 1 can chickpeas (drained and rinsed)
- Cucumber (diced)
- Cherry tomatoes (halved)
- Red onion (finely chopped)
- Feta cheese (crumbled)
- Kalamata olives
- Olive oil and lemon juice for dressing

Nutritional Components (per serving):
- Protein: 12g
- Fiber: 8g
- Healthy Fats: 10g
- Iron: 15% of daily value

Instructions:
- Combine chickpeas, cucumber, cherry tomatoes, red onion, feta cheese, and Kalamata olives in a bowl.
- Drizzle with olive oil and lemon juice.

Dinner: Teriyaki Tofu Stir-Fry with Brown Rice

Ingredients:
- 1 cup tofu (cubed)
- Mixed vegetables (broccoli, bell peppers, snap peas, carrots)
- Brown rice (cooked)
- Teriyaki sauce

Nutritional Components (per serving):
- Protein: 15g
- Fiber: 7g
- Healthy Fats: 8g
- Carbohydrates: 40g

Instructions:
- Sauté tofu in a pan until golden.
- Add mixed vegetables and stir-fry until tender.
- Pour teriyaki sauce over the tofu and vegetables.
- Serve over a bed of cooked brown rice.

Snack: Mixed Nuts

Ingredients:
- Almonds
- Walnuts
- Pistachios

Nutritional Components (per serving):
- Protein: 10g
- Fiber: 5g
- Healthy Fats: 20g
- Antioxidants

Instructions:
- Create a mix of almonds, walnuts, and pistachios for a satisfying and nutrient-packed snack.

Dessert: Coconut and Berry Nice Cream

Ingredients:
- Frozen berries
- Coconut milk

Nutritional Components (per serving):
- Fiber: 5g
- Healthy Fats: 8g
- Antioxidants: High
- Natural Sugars

Instructions:
- Blend frozen berries with coconut milk until smooth.
- Enjoy guilt-free and delicious nice cream.

Grocery List for Day 3

Chia seeds, Almond milk, Ripe mango, Canned chickpeas, Cucumber, Cherry tomatoes, Red onion, Feta cheese, Kalamata olives, Olive oil, Lemon, Tofu, Mixed vegetables (broccoli, bell peppers, snap peas, carrots), Brown rice, Teriyaki sauce, Mixed nuts (almonds, walnuts, pistachios), Frozen berries, Coconut milk.

Day 4: Fusion of Flavors

Breakfast: Acai Bowl with Tropical Fruits

Ingredients:
- Acai packets
- Banana
- Pineapple
- Mango
- Coconut flakes

Nutritional Components (per serving):
- Protein: 8g
- Fiber: 10g
- Healthy Fats: 6g
- Vitamin C: 70% of daily value

Instructions:
- Blend acai packets with banana, pineapple, and mango until smooth.
- Pour into a bowl and top with sliced banana, pineapple, mango, and coconut flakes.

Lunch: Turkey and Avocado Wrap

Ingredients:
- Whole wheat wraps
- Sliced turkey breast
- Avocado
- Lettuce
- Tomato
- Mustard

Nutritional Components (per serving):
- Protein: 18g
- Fiber: 8g
- Healthy Fats: 10g
- Vitamin A: 15% of daily value

Instructions:
- Lay out a whole wheat wrap.
- Layer sliced turkey, avocado, lettuce, tomato, and a drizzle of mustard.
- Roll it up for a delicious and satisfying wrap.

Dinner: Mexican Cauliflower Rice Bowl

Ingredients:
- Cauliflower rice
- Black beans
- Corn
- Salsa
- Avocado
- Lime

Nutritional Components (per serving):
- Protein: 10g
- Fiber: 12g
- Healthy Fats: 15g
- Vitamin C: 20% of daily value

Instructions:
- Sauté cauliflower rice until cooked.
- Mix in black beans, corn, and salsa.
- Top with sliced avocado and a squeeze of lime.

Snack: Frozen Banana Bites

Ingredients:
- Banana slices
- Dark chocolate (70% cocoa or higher)

Nutritional Components (per serving):
- Fiber: 3g
- Antioxidants: High
- Natural Sugars

Instructions:
- Slice bananas and dip each slice in melted dark chocolate.
- Allow to cool and harden for a sweet and satisfying snack.

Dessert: Peachy Green Smoothie

Ingredients:
- Handful of spinach
- Peach
- Greek yogurt
- Almond milk

Nutritional Components (per serving):
- Protein: 6g
- Fiber: 8g
- Healthy Fats: 4g
- Vitamin A: 50% of daily value

Instructions:
- Blend spinach, peach, Greek yogurt, and almond milk until smooth.

- Pour into a glass and enjoy a nutrient-packed green smoothie.

Grocery List for Day 4

Acai packets, Banana, Pineapple, Mango, Coconut flakes, Whole wheat wraps, Sliced turkey breast, Avocado, Lettuce, Tomato, Mustard, Cauliflower rice, Black beans, Corn, Salsa, Lime, Banana slices, Dark chocolate, Spinach, Peach, Greek yogurt, Almond milk

Day 5: Mediterranean Elegance

Breakfast: Mediterranean Egg White Omelette

Ingredients:
- Egg whites
- Spinach
- Feta cheese
- Tomatoes
- Olives

Nutritional Components (per serving):
- Protein: 20g
- Fiber: 4g
- Healthy Fats: 8g
- Vitamin A: 25% of daily value

Instructions:

- Whisk egg whites and pour into a hot pan.
- Add spinach, feta cheese, tomatoes, and olives.
- Fold into an omelet for a protein-packed breakfast.

Lunch: Quinoa and Chickpea Greek Salad

Ingredients:

- Quinoa
- Chickpeas
- Cucumber
- Cherry tomatoes
- Red onion
- Feta cheese
- Greek dressing

Nutritional Components (per serving):

- Protein: 15g
- Fiber: 8g
- Healthy Fats: 10g
- Vitamin C: 20% of daily value

Instructions:

- Combine cooked quinoa, chickpeas, cucumber, cherry tomatoes, red onion, and feta cheese.

- Drizzle with Greek dressing for a refreshing and nutritious salad.

Dinner: Baked Salmon with Quinoa and Asparagus

Ingredients:
- Salmon filets
- Quinoa
- Asparagus
- Lemon
- Olive oil
- Dill

Nutritional Components (per serving):
- Protein: 25g
- Fiber: 5g
- Healthy Fats: 12g
- Vitamin C: 30% of daily value

Instructions:
- Preheat the oven to 375°F (190°C).
- Season salmon with olive oil, lemon, and dill.
- Bake salmon alongside quinoa and asparagus until fully cooked.

Snack: Mediterranean Hummus Plate

Ingredients:

- Hummus
- Cherry tomatoes
- Cucumber
- Kalamata olives

Nutritional Components (per serving):

- Protein: 6g
- Fiber: 5g
- Healthy Fats: 8g

Instructions:

- Arrange hummus, cherry tomatoes, cucumber, and Kalamata olives for a delightful snack.

Dessert: Fig and Walnut Yogurt Parfait

Ingredients:

- Greek yogurt
- Figs
- Walnuts
- Honey

Nutritional Components (per serving):

- Protein: 10g
- Fiber: 5g
- Healthy Fats: 12g

Instructions:
- Layer Greek yogurt with fresh figs, walnuts, and a drizzle of honey.

Smoothie: Refreshing Citrus Smoothie

Ingredients:
- Orange
- Grapefruit
- Banana
- Coconut water

Nutritional Components (per serving):
- Vitamin C: 150% of daily value
- Fiber: 7g
- Healthy Fats: 4g

Instructions:
- Blend orange, grapefruit, banana, and coconut water until smooth.
- Enjoy a citrus-infused smoothie.

Grocery List for Day 5:

Egg whites, Spinach, Feta cheese, Tomatoes, Olives, Quinoa, Chickpeas, Cucumber, Cherry tomatoes, Red onion, Greek dressing, Salmon filets, Asparagus, Lemon, Olive oil, Dill, Hummus,

Kalamata olives, Greek yogurt, Figs, Walnuts, Honey, Orange, Grapefruit, Banana, Coconut water.

Day 6: Vibrant Variety

Breakfast: Berry and Spinach Smoothie

Ingredients:

- Mixed berries (strawberries, blueberries, raspberries)
- Spinach
- Banana
- Greek yogurt
- Almond milk

Nutritional Components (per serving):

- Protein: 12g
- Fiber: 8g
- Healthy Fats: 6g
- Vitamin C: 60% of daily value

Instructions:

- Blend mixed berries, spinach, banana, Greek yogurt, and almond milk until smooth.
- Pour into a glass and kickstart your day with a nutrient-packed smoothie.

Lunch: Caprese Salad with Balsamic Glaze

Ingredients:
- Tomatoes
- Fresh mozzarella
- Basil leaves
- Balsamic glaze
- Olive oil
- Salt and pepper to taste

Nutritional Components (per serving):
- Protein: 15g
- Calcium: 25% of daily value
- Healthy Fats: 20g
- Vitamin C: 30% of daily value

Instructions:
- Arrange sliced tomatoes, fresh mozzarella, and basil leaves on a plate.
- Drizzle with balsamic glaze and olive oil. Season with salt and pepper.

Dinner: Shrimp Stir-Fry with Vegetables and Brown Rice

Ingredients:
- Shrimp
- Mixed vegetables (broccoli, bell peppers, snap peas, carrots)

- Brown rice
- Soy sauce
- Garlic
- Ginger
- Sesame oil

Nutritional Components (per serving):
- Protein: 20g
- Fiber: 7g
- Healthy Fats: 8g
- Iron: 15% of daily value

Instructions:
- Sauté shrimp, mixed vegetables, garlic, and ginger in sesame oil.
- Add soy sauce for flavor.
- Serve over cooked brown rice for a quick and delicious stir-fry.

Snack: Almond and Cranberry Energy Bites

Ingredients:
- Almonds
- Dried cranberries
- Dates
- Chia seeds

Nutritional Components (per serving):
- Protein: 8g
- Fiber: 5g
- Healthy Fats: 10g
- Iron: 10% of daily value

Instructions:
- Blend almonds, dried cranberries, dates, and chia seeds in a food processor.
- Roll into bite-sized energy balls for a satisfying snack.

Dessert: Mango and Coconut Chia Pudding

Ingredients:
- Chia seeds
- Almond milk
- Mango
- Shredded coconut

Nutritional Components (per serving):
- Protein: 10g
- Fiber: 12g
- Healthy Fats: 8g
- Vitamin C: 40% of daily value

Instructions:
- Mix chia seeds with almond milk and refrigerate until pudding consistency.

- Top with diced mango and shredded coconut for a tropical treat.

Grocery List for Day 6:

Mixed berries, Spinach, Banana, Greek yogurt, Almond milk, Tomatoes, Fresh mozzarella, Basil leaves, Balsamic glaze, Olive oil, Shrimp, Mixed vegetables (broccoli, bell peppers, snap peas, carrots), Brown rice, Soy sauce, Garlic, Ginger, Sesame oil, Almonds, Dried cranberries, Dates, Chia seeds, Mango, Shredded coconut

Day 7: Sunday Special

Breakfast: Peanut Butter Banana Toast

Ingredients:
- Whole-grain bread
- Peanut butter
- Banana
- Honey (optional)

Nutritional Components (per serving):
- Protein: 10g
- Fiber: 6g
- Healthy Fats: 10g
- Potassium: 15% of daily value

Instructions:
- Toast whole-grain bread.
- Spread peanut butter and top with sliced banana. Drizzle with honey if desired.

Lunch: Spinach and Feta Stuffed Chicken Breast

Ingredients:
- Chicken breast
- Spinach
- Feta cheese
- Olive oil
- Lemon
- Garlic
- Salt and pepper to taste

Nutritional Components (per serving):
- Protein: 25g
- Calcium: 15% of daily value
- Healthy Fats: 12g
- Vitamin C: 30% of daily value

Instructions:
- Preheat the oven to 375°F (190°C).
- Butterfly chicken breast and stuff with spinach and feta.
- Drizzle with olive oil, lemon, and season with garlic, salt, and pepper. Bake until cooked through.

Dinner: Veggie-Packed Pasta Primavera

Ingredients:
- Whole-grain pasta
- Mixed vegetables (zucchini, cherry tomatoes, bell peppers, broccoli)
- Olive oil
- Garlic
- Parmesan cheese

Nutritional Components (per serving):
- Protein: 12g
- Fiber: 8g
- Healthy Fats: 10g
- Calcium: 20% of daily value

Instructions:
- Cook whole-grain pasta according to package instructions.
- Sauté mixed vegetables in olive oil and garlic.
- Toss pasta and vegetables together, sprinkle with Parmesan cheese.

Snack: Greek Yogurt with Berries

Ingredients:
- Greek yogurt
- Mixed berries (strawberries, blueberries, raspberries)

Nutritional Components (per serving):
- Protein: 15g
- Fiber: 5g
- Healthy Fats: 5g
- Vitamin C: 50% of daily value

Instructions:
- Spoon Greek yogurt into a bowl.
- Top with mixed berries for a simple and nutritious snack.

Dessert: Dark Chocolate-Dipped Banana Slices

Ingredients:
- Banana
- Dark chocolate (70% cocoa or higher)

Nutritional Components (per serving):
- Fiber: 4g
- Antioxidants: High
- Natural Sugars

Instructions:

- Slice bananas and dip each slice in melted dark chocolate.
- Allow to cool and harden for a sweet and satisfying dessert.

Grocery List for Day 7

Whole-grain bread, Peanut butter, Banana, Honey, Chicken breast, Spinach, Feta cheese, Olive oil, Lemon, Garlic, Salt and pepper, Whole-grain pasta, Mixed vegetables (zucchini, cherry tomatoes, bell peppers, broccoli), Parmesan cheese, Greek yogurt, Mixed berries (strawberries, blueberries, raspberries), Dark chocolate.

WEEK 2 - CULINARY HARMONY: CRAFTING DASH DIET SYMPHONIES

Here's a diverse and flavorful weekly meal plan for Week 2. Please keep in mind that the serving sizes and nutritional values are approximate and may vary based on specific ingredients and preparation methods.

Day 1: Energizing Start

Breakfast: Blueberry Oatmeal with Almond Butter

Ingredients:
- Rolled oats
- Almond milk
- Blueberries
- Almond butter
- Chia seeds

Nutritional Components (per serving):
- Protein: 10g
- Fiber: 8g
- Healthy Fats: 12g
- Antioxidants: High

Instructions:
- Cook rolled oats with almond milk.
- Top with blueberries, a dollop of almond butter, and a sprinkle of chia seeds.

Lunch: Chickpea and Avocado Salad Wrap

Ingredients:
- Whole wheat wrap
- Chickpeas (canned, drained, and rinsed)
- Avocado
- Cherry tomatoes
- Cucumber
- Lettuce
- Hummus

Nutritional Components (per serving):
- Protein: 15g
- Fiber: 10g
- Healthy Fats: 18g
- Vitamin C: 25% of daily value

Instructions:
- Spread hummus on a whole wheat wrap.
- Fill with chickpeas, sliced avocado, cherry tomatoes, cucumber, and lettuce.
- Roll it up for a delicious and filling wrap.

Dinner: Grilled Vegetable and Quinoa Bowl

Ingredients:
- Quinoa
- Zucchini
- Bell peppers (assorted colors)
- Red onion
- Cherry tomatoes
- Olive oil
- Balsamic vinegar
- Fresh basil

Nutritional Components (per serving):
- Protein: 12g
- Fiber: 8g
- Healthy Fats: 10g
- Vitamin C: 70% of daily value

Instructions:
- Cook quinoa according to package instructions.
- Grill zucchini, bell peppers, and red onion.
- Toss grilled vegetables with quinoa, cherry tomatoes, olive oil, balsamic vinegar, and fresh basil.

Snack: Cottage Cheese with Pineapple

Ingredients:
- Cottage cheese
- Fresh pineapple

Nutritional Components (per serving):
- Protein: 15g
- Vitamin C: 60% of daily value
- Calcium: 20% of daily value

Instructions:
- Combine cottage cheese with fresh pineapple for a protein-packed and refreshing snack.

Dessert: Dark Chocolate-Covered Almonds

Ingredients:
- Dark chocolate (70% cocoa or higher)
- Almonds

Nutritional Components (per serving):
- Protein: 8g
- Fiber: 5g
- Healthy Fats: 15g
- Antioxidants: High

Instructions:
- Melt dark chocolate and dip almonds into the chocolate.
- Allow to cool and harden for a sweet and satisfying dessert.

Grocery List for Day 1

Rolled oats, Almond milk, Blueberries, Almond butter, Chia seeds, Whole wheat wraps, Chickpeas, Avocado, Cherry tomatoes, Cucumber, Lettuce, Hummus, Quinoa, Zucchini, Bell peppers (assorted colors), Red onion, Olive oil, Balsamic vinegar, Fresh basil, Cottage cheese, Fresh pineapple, Dark chocolate, Almonds

Day 2: Wholesome Choices

Breakfast: Greek Yogurt Parfait with Mixed Berries

Ingredients:
- Greek yogurt
- Mixed berries (strawberries, blueberries, raspberries)
- Granola
- Honey

Nutritional Components (per serving):
- Protein: 15g

- Fiber: 8g
- Healthy Fats: 5g
- Antioxidants: High

Instructions:
- Layer Greek yogurt with mixed berries and granola.
- Drizzle with honey for added sweetness.

Lunch: Quinoa and Black Bean Stuffed Bell Peppers

Ingredients:
- Bell peppers (assorted colors)
- Quinoa
- Black beans (canned, drained, and rinsed)
- Corn kernels
- Salsa
- Avocado

Nutritional Components (per serving):
- Protein: 14g
- Fiber: 10g
- Healthy Fats: 8g
- Vitamin C: 120% of daily value

Instructions:
- Cook quinoa according to package instructions.

- Mix quinoa with black beans, corn, and salsa.
- Stuff bell peppers with the quinoa mixture and top with sliced avocado.

Dinner: Teriyaki Chicken Stir-Fry with Brown Rice

Ingredients:
- Chicken breast
- Mixed vegetables (broccoli, bell peppers, snap peas, carrots)
- Brown rice
- Teriyaki sauce
- Sesame seeds

Nutritional Components (per serving):
- Protein: 20g
- Fiber: 7g
- Healthy Fats: 6g
- Iron: 15% of daily value

Instructions:
- Sauté chicken breast and mixed vegetables in a pan.
- Add teriyaki sauce and cook until chicken is thoroughly cooked.
- Serve over brown rice and sprinkle with sesame seeds.

Snack: Apple Slices with Almond Butter

Ingredients:
- Apple (sliced)
- Almond butter

Nutritional Components (per serving):
- Protein: 4g
- Fiber: 6g
- Healthy Fats: 10g
- Vitamin C: 8% of daily value

Instructions:
- Slice the apple and spread almond butter on each slice for a satisfying snack.

Dessert: Mango Coconut Chia Popsicles

Ingredients:
- Chia seeds
- Coconut milk
- Mango (pureed)

Nutritional Components (per serving):
- Protein: 6g
- Fiber: 8g
- Healthy Fats: 10g
- Vitamin C: 60% of daily value

Instructions:
- Mix chia seeds with coconut milk and let it sit until it thickens.
- Layer chia mixture with mango puree in popsicle molds and freeze.

Grocery List for Day 2

Greek yogurt, Mixed berries (strawberries, blueberries, raspberries), Granola, Honey, Bell peppers (assorted colors), Quinoa, Black beans, Corn kernels, Salsa, Avocado, Chicken breast, Mixed vegetables (broccoli, bell peppers, snap peas, carrots), Brown rice, Teriyaki sauce, Sesame seeds, Apple, Almond butter, Chia seeds, Coconut milk, Mango.

Day 3: Fusion of Flavors

Breakfast: Banana and Spinach Smoothie Bowl

Ingredients:
- Banana
- Spinach
- Greek yogurt
- Almond milk
- Toppings: Sliced almonds, chia seeds, sliced strawberries

Nutritional Components (per serving):
- Protein: 12g
- Fiber: 8g
- Healthy Fats: 6g
- Vitamin C: 70% of daily value

Instructions:
- Blend banana, spinach, Greek yogurt, and almond milk until smooth.
- Pour into a bowl and top with sliced almonds, chia seeds, and sliced strawberries.

Lunch: Lentil and Vegetable Stew

Ingredients:
- Lentils
- Carrots
- Celery
- Onion
- Garlic
- Vegetable broth
- Tomatoes
- Spinach

Nutritional Components (per serving):
- Protein: 15g
- Fiber: 10g
- Healthy Fats: 4g
- Iron: 20% of daily value

Instructions:
- Sauté onions and garlic, add lentils, carrots, celery, tomatoes, and vegetable broth.
- Simmer until lentils are tender, then stir in spinach.

Dinner: Baked Cod with Lemon and Herbs

Ingredients:
- Cod filets
- Lemon
- Fresh herbs (parsley, dill)
- Olive oil
- Garlic
- Salt and pepper to taste

Nutritional Components (per serving):
- Protein: 25g
- Healthy Fats: 10g
- Vitamin C: 30% of daily value

Instructions:
- Preheat the oven to 400°F (200°C).
- Place cod filets on a baking sheet, drizzle with olive oil, lemon juice, minced garlic, fresh herbs, salt, and pepper.
- Bake until the fish is cooked through and flakes easily.

Snack: Yogurt and Berry Parfait

Ingredients:
- Greek yogurt
- Mixed berries (blueberries, raspberries)
- Granola

Nutritional Components (per serving):
- Protein: 10g
- Fiber: 5g
- Healthy Fats: 8g

Instructions:
- Layer Greek yogurt with mixed berries and granola for a delightful snack.

Dessert: Chocolate Avocado Mousse

Ingredients:
- Ripe avocados
- Cocoa powder
- Maple syrup
- Vanilla extract

Nutritional Components (per serving):
- Protein: 8g
- Fiber: 10g
- Healthy Fats: 15g

- Antioxidants: High

Instructions:
- Blend ripe avocados, cocoa powder, maple syrup, and vanilla extract until smooth.
- Chill in the refrigerator before serving.

Grocery List for Day 3:
Banana, Spinach, Greek yogurt, Almond milk, Sliced almonds, Chia seeds, Strawberries, Lentils, Carrots, Celery, Onion, Garlic, Vegetable broth, Tomatoes, Fresh herbs (parsley, dill), Cod filets, Lemon, Olive oil, Salt and pepper, Mixed berries (blueberries, raspberries), Granola, Ripe avocados, Cocoa powder, Maple syrup, Vanilla extract.

Day 4: Fresh and Flavorful

Breakfast: Spinach and Feta Egg Muffins

Ingredients:
- Eggs
- Spinach
- Feta cheese
- Cherry tomatoes
- Salt and pepper to taste

Nutritional Components (per serving):

- Protein: 15g
- Fiber: 5g
- Healthy Fats: 10g
- Vitamin A: 30% of daily value

Instructions:

- Whisk eggs and mix with chopped spinach, crumbled feta, and halved cherry tomatoes.
- Pour into muffin cups and bake until eggs are set.

Lunch: Quinoa Salad with Roasted Vegetables

Ingredients:

- Quinoa
- Mixed vegetables (zucchini, bell peppers, cherry tomatoes)
- Olive oil
- Balsamic vinegar
- Fresh basil
- Feta cheese (optional)

Nutritional Components (per serving):

- Protein: 12g
- Fiber: 8g
- Healthy Fats: 10g
- Vitamin C: 50% of daily value

Instructions:

- Cook quinoa according to package instructions.
- Roast mixed vegetables with olive oil and balsamic vinegar.
- Toss quinoa with roasted vegetables, fresh basil, and optional feta cheese.

Dinner: Thai Coconut Curry with Tofu and Vegetables

Ingredients:

- Tofu
- Mixed vegetables (broccoli, bell peppers, carrots)
- Coconut milk
- Red curry paste
- Soy sauce
- Brown rice

Nutritional Components (per serving):

- Protein: 18g
- Fiber: 6g
- Healthy Fats: 15g
- Iron: 20% of daily value

Instructions:

- Sauté tofu and mixed vegetables in a pan.
- Add coconut milk, red curry paste, and soy sauce. Simmer until vegetables are tender.
- Serve over brown rice.

Snack: Greek Yogurt with Cucumber and Dill

Ingredients:

- Greek yogurt
- Cucumber
- Fresh dill

Nutritional Components (per serving):

- Protein: 10g
- Fiber: 3g
- Healthy Fats: 6g

Instructions:

- Mix Greek yogurt with diced cucumber and chopped fresh dill for a refreshing snack.

Dessert: Mixed Berry Sorbet

Ingredients:

- Mixed berries (strawberries, blueberries, raspberries)
- Honey or maple syrup (optional)
- Lemon juice

Nutritional Components (per serving):
- Fiber: 5g
- Antioxidants: High
- Natural Sugars

Instructions:
- Blend mixed berries with honey or maple syrup (optional) and lemon juice.
- Freeze the mixture and blend again until smooth for a delightful sorbet.

Grocery List for Day 4:

Eggs, Spinach, Feta cheese, Cherry tomatoes, Quinoa, Mixed vegetables (zucchini, bell peppers, cherry tomatoes), Olive oil, Balsamic vinegar, Fresh basil, Feta cheese (optional), Tofu, Mixed vegetables (broccoli, bell peppers, carrots), Coconut milk, Red curry paste, Soy sauce, Brown rice, Greek yogurt, Cucumber, Fresh dill, Mixed berries (strawberries, blueberries, raspberries), Honey or maple syrup, Lemon juice.

Day 5: Vibrant and Satisfying

Breakfast: Berry and Banana Smoothie Bowl
Ingredients:
- Mixed berries (strawberries, blueberries, raspberries)

- Banana
- Greek yogurt
- Almond milk
- Toppings: Sliced almonds, chia seeds, shredded coconut

Nutritional Components (per serving):
- Protein: 12g
- Fiber: 8g
- Healthy Fats: 6g
- Vitamin C: 80% of daily value

Instructions:
- Blend mixed berries, banana, Greek yogurt, and almond milk until smooth.
- Pour into a bowl and top with sliced almonds, chia seeds, and shredded coconut.

Lunch: Chickpea and Spinach Salad with Lemon Tahini Dressing

Ingredients:
- Chickpeas (canned, drained, and rinsed)
- Spinach
- Cherry tomatoes
- Cucumber
- Red onion
- Feta cheese
- Lemon tahini dressing

Nutritional Components (per serving):
- Protein: 14g
- Fiber: 8g
- Healthy Fats: 10g
- Vitamin C: 40% of daily value

Instructions:
- Combine chickpeas, spinach, cherry tomatoes, cucumber, red onion, and feta cheese.
- Drizzle with lemon tahini dressing for a flavorful salad.

Dinner: Grilled Salmon with Quinoa and Asparagus

Ingredients:
- Salmon filets
- Quinoa
- Asparagus
- Lemon
- Olive oil
- Dill
- Salt and pepper to taste

Nutritional Components (per serving):
- Protein: 25g
- Fiber: 5g
- Healthy Fats: 12g

- Vitamin C: 30% of daily value

Instructions:
- Season salmon with olive oil, lemon, dill, salt, and pepper.
- Grill or bake salmon alongside quinoa and asparagus until fully cooked.

Snack: Cottage Cheese with Pineapple and Walnuts

Ingredients:
- Cottage cheese
- Fresh pineapple
- Walnuts

Nutritional Components (per serving):
- Protein: 15g
- Fiber: 3g
- Healthy Fats: 10g

Instructions:
- Combine cottage cheese with fresh pineapple and top with walnuts for a satisfying snack.

Dessert: Chocolate Banana Chia Pudding
Ingredients:
- Chia seeds
- Almond milk

- Cocoa powder
- Banana

Nutritional Components (per serving):
- Protein: 8g
- Fiber: 10g
- Healthy Fats: 6g
- Vitamin C: 15% of daily value

Instructions:
- Mix chia seeds with almond milk, cocoa powder, and mashed banana.
- Refrigerate until the mixture thickens into a pudding-like consistency.

Grocery List for Day 5:

Mixed berries (strawberries, blueberries, raspberries), Banana, Greek yogurt, Almond milk, Sliced almonds, Chia seeds, Shredded coconut, Chickpeas, Spinach, Cherry tomatoes, Cucumber, Red onion, Feta cheese, Lemon tahini dressing, Salmon filets, Quinoa, Asparagus, Lemon, Olive oil, Dill, Cottage cheese, Fresh pineapple, Walnuts, Chia seeds, Cocoa powder

Day 6: Wholesome Delights

Breakfast: Avocado Toast with Poached Eggs

Ingredients:
- Whole-grain bread
- Avocado
- Eggs
- Salt and pepper to taste
- Optional toppings: Cherry tomatoes, red pepper flakes

Nutritional Components (per serving):
- Protein: 15g
- Fiber: 8g
- Healthy Fats: 12g
- Vitamin C: 20% of daily value

Instructions:
- Toast whole-grain bread and spread avocado.
- Top with poached eggs and season with salt and pepper. Add optional toppings if desired.

Lunch: Quinoa and Kale Salad with Lemon Vinaigrette

Ingredients:
- Quinoa
- Kale
- Cherry tomatoes
- Avocado
- Feta cheese
- Pumpkin seeds
- Lemon vinaigrette dressing

Nutritional Components (per serving):
- Protein: 12g
- Fiber: 8g
- Healthy Fats: 10g
- Vitamin C: 40% of daily value

Instructions:
- Cook quinoa according to package instructions.
- Combine quinoa with chopped kale, cherry tomatoes, diced avocado, feta cheese, and pumpkin seeds.
- Drizzle with lemon vinaigrette dressing for a refreshing salad.

Dinner: Turkey and Vegetable Stir-Fry with Brown Rice

Ingredients:
- Ground turkey
- Mixed vegetables (broccoli, bell peppers, snap peas, carrots)
- Brown rice
- Soy sauce
- Garlic
- Ginger
- Sesame oil

Nutritional Components (per serving):
- Protein: 20g
- Fiber: 7g
- Healthy Fats: 8g
- Iron: 15% of daily value

Instructions:
- Sauté ground turkey and mixed vegetables in a pan.
- Add soy sauce, minced garlic, ginger, and a drizzle of sesame oil.
- Serve over cooked brown rice for a flavorful stir-fry.

Snack: Apple Slices with Peanut Butter

Ingredients:
- Apple (sliced)
- Peanut butter

Nutritional Components (per serving):
- Protein: 4g
- Fiber: 6g
- Healthy Fats: 10g
- Vitamin C: 8% of daily value

Instructions:
- Slice the apple and spread peanut butter on each slice for a satisfying snack.

Dessert: Mixed Berry and Yogurt Popsicles

Ingredients:
- Mixed berries (strawberries, blueberries, raspberries)
- Greek yogurt
- Honey

Nutritional Components (per serving):
- Protein: 6g
- Fiber: 5g
- Healthy Fats: 4g
- Vitamin C: 50% of daily value

Instructions:
- Blend mixed berries with Greek yogurt and honey.
- Pour into popsicle molds and freeze for a delightful treat.

Grocery List for Day 6:

Whole-grain bread, Avocado, Eggs, Cherry tomatoes, Red pepper flakes, Quinoa, Kale, Avocado, Feta cheese, Pumpkin seeds, Lemon vinaigrette dressing, Ground turkey, Mixed vegetables (broccoli, bell peppers, snap peas, carrots), Brown rice, Soy sauce, Garlic, Ginger, Sesame oil, Apple, Peanut butter, Mixed berries (strawberries, blueberries, raspberries), Greek yogurt, Honey

Day 7: Culmination of Flavor

Breakfast: Spinach and Mushroom Omelette

Ingredients:
- Eggs
- Spinach
- Mushrooms
- Feta cheese
- Olive oil

- Salt and pepper to taste

Nutritional Components (per serving):
- Protein: 15g
- Fiber: 5g
- Healthy Fats: 10g
- Vitamin A: 25% of daily value

Instructions:
- Sauté spinach and mushrooms in olive oil until wilted.
- Pour beaten eggs over the vegetables, add crumbled feta cheese, and cook until the eggs are set.

Lunch: Mediterranean Chickpea Bowl

Ingredients:
- Chickpeas (canned, drained, and rinsed)
- Cherry tomatoes
- Cucumber
- Kalamata olives
- Red onion
- Feta cheese
- Olive oil
- Lemon juice
- Fresh oregano

Nutritional Components (per serving):
- Protein: 14g
- Fiber: 8g
- Healthy Fats: 12g
- Vitamin C: 30% of daily value

Instructions:
- Combine chickpeas, cherry tomatoes, cucumber, Kalamata olives, red onion, and feta cheese.
- Drizzle with olive oil, lemon juice, and sprinkle with fresh oregano.

Dinner: Shrimp and Vegetable Stir-Fry with Quinoa

Ingredients:
- Shrimp
- Mixed vegetables (bell peppers, broccoli, snap peas, carrots)
- Quinoa
- Soy sauce
- Garlic
- Ginger
- Sesame oil

Nutritional Components (per serving):
- Protein: 20g
- Fiber: 7g
- Healthy Fats: 8g

- Iron: 15% of daily value

Instructions:
- Sauté shrimp and mixed vegetables in a pan.
- Add soy sauce, minced garlic, ginger, and a drizzle of sesame oil.
- Serve over cooked quinoa for a quick and tasty stir-fry.

Snack: Hummus with Sliced Bell Peppers

Ingredients:
- Hummus
- Bell peppers (assorted colors)

Nutritional Components (per serving):
- Protein: 6g
- Fiber: 5g
- Healthy Fats: 8g
- Vitamin C: 150% of daily value

Instructions:
- Dip assorted bell pepper slices into hummus for a satisfying and nutritious snack.

Dessert: Tropical Fruit Salad with Mint
Ingredients:
- Pineapple
- Mango

- Kiwi
- Fresh mint leaves

Nutritional Components (per serving):
- Fiber: 6g
- Vitamin C: 150% of daily value
- Antioxidants: High

Instructions:
- Dice pineapple, mango, and kiwi.
- Toss together and garnish with fresh mint leaves for a refreshing fruit salad.

Grocery List for Day 7:
Eggs, Spinach, Mushrooms, Feta cheese, Olive oil, Chickpeas, Cherry tomatoes, Cucumber, Kalamata olives, Red onion, Feta cheese, Olive oil, Lemon juice, Fresh oregano, Shrimp, Mixed vegetables (bell peppers, broccoli, snap peas, carrots), Quinoa, Soy sauce, Garlic, Ginger, Sesame oil, Hummus, Bell peppers (assorted colors), Pineapple, Mango, Kiwi, Fresh mint leaves.

WEEK 3 - VIBRANT VARIETY: A DASH DIET PALETTE OF HEALTHY CHOICES

Let's continue with a diverse and flavorful meal plan for Week 3. Keep in mind that serving sizes and nutritional values are approximate and may vary based on specific ingredients and preparation methods.

Day 1: Energizing Choices

Breakfast: Blueberry and Almond Overnight Oats

Ingredients:
- Rolled oats
- Almond milk
- Blueberries
- Almonds (sliced)
- Chia seeds

Nutritional Components (per serving):
- Protein: 10g
- Fiber: 8g
- Healthy Fats: 12g
- Antioxidants: High

Instructions:

- Combine rolled oats, almond milk, blueberries, sliced almonds, and chia seeds in a jar.
- Refrigerate overnight and enjoy a quick, nutritious breakfast.

Lunch: Quinoa and Black Bean Wrap

Ingredients:

- Quinoa
- Black beans (canned, drained, and rinsed)
- Avocado
- Cherry tomatoes
- Spinach
- Whole-grain wrap

Nutritional Components (per serving):
- Protein: 15g
- Fiber: 10g
- Healthy Fats: 18g
- Vitamin C: 25% of daily value

Instructions:
- Mix quinoa with black beans, avocado, cherry tomatoes, and spinach.
- Fill a whole-grain wrap with the mixture for a satisfying lunch.

Dinner: Baked Chicken Breast with Sweet Potato and Broccoli

Ingredients:
- Chicken breast
- Sweet potatoes
- Broccoli
- Olive oil
- Garlic powder
- Paprika
- Salt and pepper to taste

Nutritional Components (per serving):
- Protein: 25g
- Fiber: 7g
- Healthy Fats: 8g
- Vitamin C: 90% of daily value

Instructions:
- Season chicken breast with garlic powder, paprika, salt, and pepper.
- Bake alongside sweet potatoes and broccoli, drizzled with olive oil.

Snack: Greek Yogurt with Berries
Ingredients:
- Greek yogurt

- Mixed berries (strawberries, blueberries, raspberries)

Nutritional Components (per serving):
- Protein: 10g
- Fiber: 5g
- Healthy Fats: 8g

Instructions:
- Top Greek yogurt with mixed berries for a quick and protein-packed snack.

Dessert: Dark Chocolate and Walnut Energy Bites

Ingredients:
- Dates (pitted)
- Walnuts
- Dark chocolate (70% cocoa or higher)
- Chia seeds

Nutritional Components (per serving):
- Protein: 8g
- Fiber: 6g
- Healthy Fats: 10g
- Antioxidants: High

Instructions:
- Blend dates, walnuts, dark chocolate, and chia seeds in a food processor.

- Roll into small energy bites for a sweet treat.

Grocery List for Day 1:
Rolled oats, Almond milk, Blueberries, Almonds (sliced), Chia seeds, Quinoa, Black beans (canned), Avocado, Cherry tomatoes, Spinach, Whole-grain wraps, Chicken breast, Sweet potatoes, Broccoli, Olive oil, Garlic powder, Paprika, Salt and pepper, Greek yogurt, Mixed berries (strawberries, blueberries, raspberries), Dates, Walnuts, Dark chocolate (70% cocoa or higher).

Day 2: Flavorful and Balanced

Breakfast: Banana and Peanut Butter Smoothie

Ingredients:
- Bananas
- Peanut butter
- Greek yogurt
- Almond milk
- Ice cubes

Nutritional Components (per serving):
- Protein: 12g
- Fiber: 5g
- Healthy Fats: 10g
- Potassium: High

Instructions:

- Blend bananas, peanut butter, Greek yogurt, almond milk, and ice cubes until smooth.
- Enjoy a creamy and energizing smoothie to kickstart your day.

Lunch: Chickpea and Avocado Salad

Ingredients:

- Chickpeas (canned, drained, and rinsed)
- Avocado
- Cherry tomatoes
- Cucumber
- Red onion
- Feta cheese
- Olive oil
- Lemon juice
- Fresh basil

Nutritional Components (per serving):

- Protein: 14g
- Fiber: 8g
- Healthy Fats: 15g
- Vitamin C: 30% of daily value

Instructions:

- Combine chickpeas, diced avocado, cherry tomatoes, cucumber, red onion, and crumbled feta cheese.
- Drizzle with olive oil, lemon juice, and garnish with fresh basil for a delightful salad.

Dinner: Vegetarian Stir-Fry with Tofu and Brown Rice

Ingredients:
- Tofu
- Mixed vegetables (bell peppers, broccoli, carrots, snap peas)
- Brown rice
- Soy sauce
- Garlic
- Ginger
- Sesame oil

Nutritional Components (per serving):
- Protein: 18g
- Fiber: 8g
- Healthy Fats: 10g
- Iron: 15% of daily value

Instructions:
- Sauté tofu and mixed vegetables in a pan.

- Add soy sauce, minced garlic, ginger, and a drizzle of sesame oil.
- Serve over cooked brown rice for a quick and tasty stir-fry.

Snack: Apple and Almond Butter Rice Cakes

Ingredients:
- Rice cakes
- Almond butter
- Apple (sliced)

Nutritional Components (per serving):
- Protein: 6g
- Fiber: 4g
- Healthy Fats: 8g
- Vitamin C: 10% of daily value

Instructions:
- Spread almond butter on rice cakes and top with sliced apple for a satisfying snack.

Dessert: Berry Parfait with Greek Yogurt

Ingredients:
- Mixed berries (strawberries, blueberries, raspberries)
- Greek yogurt
- Granola

Nutritional Components (per serving):
- Protein: 10g
- Fiber: 6g
- Healthy Fats: 8g
- Antioxidants: High

Instructions:
- Layer Greek yogurt with mixed berries and granola for a delightful and healthy dessert.

Grocery List for Day 2:

Bananas, Peanut butter, Greek yogurt, Almond milk, Ice cubes, Chickpeas (canned), Avocado, Cherry tomatoes, Cucumber, Red onion, Feta cheese, Olive oil, Lemon juice, Fresh basil, Tofu, Mixed vegetables (bell peppers, broccoli, carrots, snap peas), Brown rice, Soy sauce, Garlic, Ginger, Sesame oil, Rice cakes, Almond butter, Apple, Mixed berries (strawberries, blueberries, raspberries), Granola.

Day 3: Wholesome Choices

Breakfast: Spinach and Mushroom Breakfast Burrito

Ingredients:
- Whole-grain tortilla

- Eggs
- Spinach
- Mushrooms
- Feta cheese
- Salsa

Nutritional Components (per serving):
- Protein: 15g
- Fiber: 5g
- Healthy Fats: 10g
- Vitamin A: 20% of daily value

Instructions:
- Scramble eggs and sauté spinach and mushrooms.
- Fill a whole-grain tortilla with the eggs, spinach, mushrooms, crumbled feta cheese, and salsa.

Lunch: Mediterranean Quinoa Bowl

Ingredients:
- Quinoa
- Chickpeas (canned, drained, and rinsed)
- Cherry tomatoes
- Cucumber
- Kalamata olives
- Red onion
- Feta cheese

- Olive oil
- Lemon juice
- Fresh oregano

Nutritional Components (per serving):
- Protein: 14g
- Fiber: 8g
- Healthy Fats: 12g
- Vitamin C: 30% of daily value

Instructions:
- Cook quinoa according to package instructions.
- Combine quinoa with chickpeas, cherry tomatoes, cucumber, Kalamata olives, red onion, and feta cheese.
- Drizzle with olive oil, lemon juice, and sprinkle with fresh oregano.

Dinner: Grilled Vegetable and Chickpea Salad

Ingredients:
- Mixed vegetables (zucchini, bell peppers, cherry tomatoes)
- Chickpeas (canned, drained, and rinsed)
- Olive oil
- Balsamic vinegar
- Fresh basil
- Feta cheese (optional)

Nutritional Components (per serving):

- Protein: 12g
- Fiber: 8g
- Healthy Fats: 10g
- Vitamin C: 80% of daily value

Instructions:

- Grill mixed vegetables and toss with chickpeas.
- Drizzle with olive oil and balsamic vinegar, and top with fresh basil and optional feta cheese.

Snack: Cottage Cheese with Pineapple

Ingredients:

- Cottage cheese
- Fresh pineapple

Nutritional Components (per serving):

- Protein: 15g
- Fiber: 3g
- Healthy Fats: 6g

Instructions:

- Combine cottage cheese with fresh pineapple for a protein-rich and refreshing snack.

Dessert: Mango and Coconut Chia Pudding

Ingredients:
- Chia seeds
- Coconut milk
- Mango (pureed)

Nutritional Components (per serving):
- Protein: 8g
- Fiber: 10g
- Healthy Fats: 12g
- Vitamin C: 60% of daily value

Instructions:
- Mix chia seeds with coconut milk and layer with mango puree.
- Refrigerate until the mixture thickens into a delicious chia pudding.

Grocery List for Day 3:
Whole-grain tortilla, Eggs, Spinach, Mushrooms, Feta cheese, Salsa, Quinoa, Chickpeas (canned), Cherry tomatoes, Cucumber, Kalamata olives, Red onion, Feta cheese, Olive oil, Lemon juice, Fresh oregano, Mixed vegetables (zucchini, bell peppers,

cherry tomatoes), Chickpeas (canned), Balsamic vinegar, Fresh basil, Cottage cheese, Fresh pineapple, Chia seeds, Coconut milk, Mango.

Day 4: Nutrient-Rich Choices

Breakfast: Berry and Spinach Smoothie

Ingredients:
- Mixed berries (strawberries, blueberries, raspberries)
- Spinach
- Greek yogurt
- Almond milk
- Flaxseeds

Nutritional Components (per serving):
- Protein: 12g
- Fiber: 7g
- Healthy Fats: 8g
- Antioxidants: High

Instructions:
- Blend mixed berries, spinach, Greek yogurt, almond milk, and flaxseeds until smooth.
- Sip on a nutrient-packed smoothie to start your day.

Lunch: Lentil and Vegetable Wrap

Ingredients:

- Lentils (cooked)
- Whole-grain wrap
- Hummus
- Cherry tomatoes
- Cucumber
- Red onion
- Spinach

Nutritional Components (per serving):

- Protein: 14g
- Fiber: 10g
- Healthy Fats: 8g
- Iron: 25% of daily value

Instructions:

- Spread hummus on a whole-grain wrap and fill with cooked lentils, cherry tomatoes, cucumber, red onion, and spinach.
- Roll up the wrap for a satisfying and nutritious lunch.

Dinner: Baked Salmon with Quinoa and Asparagus

Ingredients:

- Salmon filets
- Quinoa
- Asparagus

- Lemon
- Olive oil
- Dill
- Salt and pepper to taste

Nutritional Components (per serving):
- Protein: 25g
- Fiber: 7g
- Healthy Fats: 12g
- Vitamin C: 30% of daily value

Instructions:
- Season salmon with olive oil, lemon, dill, salt, and pepper.
- Bake alongside quinoa and asparagus until fully cooked.

Snack: Greek Yogurt with Walnuts and Honey

Ingredients:
- Greek yogurt
- Walnuts
- Honey

Nutritional Components (per serving):
- Protein: 10g
- Fiber: 3g
- Healthy Fats: 10g

Instructions:

- Top Greek yogurt with walnuts and drizzle with honey for a delightful snack.

Dessert: Chocolate Avocado Mousse

Ingredients:

- Avocado
- Cocoa powder
- Maple syrup or honey
- Vanilla extract
- Almond milk

Nutritional Components (per serving):

- Protein: 6g
- Fiber: 7g
- Healthy Fats: 12g
- Antioxidants: High

Instructions:

- Blend avocado, cocoa powder, maple syrup or honey, vanilla extract, and almond milk until smooth.
- Chill in the refrigerator for a few hours before serving.

Grocery List for Day 4:

Mixed berries (strawberries, blueberries, raspberries), Spinach, Greek yogurt, Almond milk,

Flaxseeds, Lentils (cooked), Whole-grain wraps, Hummus, Cherry tomatoes, Cucumber, Red onion, Salmon filets, Quinoa, Asparagus, Lemon, Olive oil, Dill, Walnuts, Honey, Avocado, Cocoa powder, Maple syrup or honey, Vanilla extract.

Day 5: Tasty and Wholesome

Breakfast: Peach and Almond Overnight Oats

Ingredients:
- Rolled oats
- Almond milk
- Peaches (sliced)
- Almonds (sliced)
- Chia seeds

Nutritional Components (per serving):
- Protein: 10g
- Fiber: 8g
- Healthy Fats: 12g
- Vitamin C: 15% of daily value

Instructions:
- Combine rolled oats, almond milk, sliced peaches, sliced almonds, and chia seeds in a jar.

- Refrigerate overnight for a refreshing and nutritious breakfast.

Lunch: Caprese Salad with Quinoa

Ingredients:
- Quinoa
- Cherry tomatoes
- Fresh mozzarella
- Basil leaves
- Balsamic glaze
- Olive oil
- Salt and pepper to taste

Nutritional Components (per serving):
- Protein: 12g
- Fiber: 5g
- Healthy Fats: 10g
- Vitamin C: 25% of daily value

Instructions:
- Cook quinoa according to package instructions.
- Combine quinoa with halved cherry tomatoes, fresh mozzarella, and basil leaves.
- Drizzle with olive oil and balsamic glaze, and season with salt and pepper.

Dinner: Grilled Chicken and Vegetable Skewers
Ingredients:
- Chicken breast (cut into cubes)
- Bell peppers (assorted colors)
- Red onion
- Zucchini
- Cherry tomatoes
- Olive oil
- Lemon juice
- Garlic
- Oregano
- Salt and pepper to taste

Nutritional Components (per serving):
- Protein: 20g
- Fiber: 6g
- Healthy Fats: 8g
- Vitamin C: 80% of daily value

Instructions:
- Marinate chicken cubes in olive oil, lemon juice, minced garlic, oregano, salt, and pepper.
- Thread chicken and assorted vegetables onto skewers and grill until fully cooked.

Snack: Banana and Almond Butter Rice Cakes

Ingredients:

- Rice cakes
- Almond butter
- Banana (sliced)

Nutritional Components (per serving):
- Protein: 6g
- Fiber: 4g
- Healthy Fats: 8g
- Vitamin C: 10% of daily value

Instructions:
- Spread almond butter on rice cakes and top with sliced banana for a satisfying snack.

Dessert: Raspberry Chia Seed Pudding

Ingredients:
- Chia seeds
- Almond milk
- Raspberries

Nutritional Components (per serving):
- Protein: 8g
- Fiber: 10g
- Healthy Fats: 12g
- Antioxidants: High

Instructions:

- Mix chia seeds with almond milk and layer with mashed raspberries.
- Refrigerate until the mixture thickens into a delightful chia seed pudding.

Grocery List for Day 5:
Rolled oats, Almond milk, Peaches, Almonds (sliced), Chia seeds, Quinoa, Cherry tomatoes, Fresh mozzarella, Basil leaves, Balsamic glaze, Olive oil, Salt and pepper, Chicken breast, Bell peppers (assorted colors), Red onion, Zucchini, Cherry tomatoes, Lemon, Garlic, Oregano, Rice cakes, Almond butter, Banana, Raspberries.

Day 6: Culmination of Delights

Breakfast: Mango and Coconut Smoothie Bowl

Ingredients:
- Mango (frozen chunks)
- Coconut milk
- Greek yogurt
- Granola
- Shredded coconut
- Chia seeds

Nutritional Components (per serving):
- Protein: 12g

- Fiber: 8g
- Healthy Fats: 10g
- Vitamin C: 100% of daily value

Instructions:
- Blend frozen mango chunks, coconut milk, and Greek yogurt until smooth.
- Pour into a bowl and top with granola, shredded coconut, and chia seeds for a tropical delight.

Lunch: Sweet Potato and Black Bean Salad

Ingredients:
- Sweet potatoes (roasted)
- Black beans (canned, drained, and rinsed)
- Corn kernels (fresh or frozen)
- Avocado
- Lime
- Cilantro
- Olive oil
- Cumin
- Salt and pepper to taste

Nutritional Components (per serving):
- Protein: 14g
- Fiber: 10g
- Healthy Fats: 15g

- Vitamin A: 150% of daily value

Instructions:
- Roast sweet potatoes and let them cool.
- Mix sweet potatoes with black beans, corn kernels, diced avocado, lime juice, chopped cilantro, olive oil, cumin, salt, and pepper.

Dinner: Quinoa-stuffed Bell Peppers

Ingredients:
- Quinoa
- Bell peppers (assorted colors)
- Ground turkey
- Black beans (canned, drained, and rinsed)
- Corn kernels (fresh or frozen)
- Onion
- Garlic
- Tomato sauce
- Cumin
- Chili powder
- Paprika
- Shredded cheese

Nutritional Components (per serving):
- Protein: 20g

- Fiber: 8g
- Healthy Fats: 10g
- Vitamin C: 200% of daily value

Instructions:
- Cook quinoa according to package instructions.
- Sauté ground turkey, onion, and garlic. Mix with cooked quinoa, black beans, corn kernels, tomato sauce, cumin, chili powder, and paprika.
- Cut bell peppers in half, stuff with the quinoa mixture, and top with shredded cheese. Bake until the cheese is melted and bubbly.

Snack: Hummus With Carrot Sticks

Ingredients:
- Hummus
- Carrot sticks

Nutritional Components (per serving):
- Protein: 6g
- Fiber: 5g
- Healthy Fats: 8g
- Vitamin A: 300% of daily value

Instructions:
- Dip carrot sticks into hummus for a nutritious and satisfying snack.

Dessert: Mixed Berry Sorbet

Ingredients:
- Mixed berries (strawberries, blueberries, raspberries)
- Maple syrup or honey
- Lemon juice
- Fresh mint leaves

Nutritional Components (per serving):
- Fiber: 6g
- Vitamin C: 150% of daily value
- Antioxidants: High

Instructions:
- Blend mixed berries with maple syrup or honey and lemon juice until smooth.
- Freeze and scoop into bowls, garnishing with fresh mint leaves.

Grocery List For Day 6:
Mango (frozen chunks), Coconut milk, Greek yogurt, Granola, Shredded coconut, Chia seeds, Sweet potatoes, Black beans (canned), Corn kernels

(fresh or frozen), Avocado, Lime, Cilantro, Olive oil, Cumin, Salt and pepper, Quinoa, Bell peppers (assorted colors), Ground turkey, Onion, Garlic, Tomato sauce, Chili powder, Paprika, Shredded cheese, Hummus, Carrot sticks, Mixed berries (strawberries, blueberries, raspberries), Maple syrup or honey, Lemon, Fresh mint leaves.

Day 7: Energizing Choices

Breakfast: Banana and Spinach Protein Smoothie

Ingredients:
- Bananas
- Spinach
- Protein powder (of your choice)
- Almond milk
- Ice cubes

Nutritional Components (per serving):
- Protein: 15g
- Fiber: 6g
- Healthy Fats: 8g
- Potassium: High

Instructions:
- Blend bananas, spinach, protein powder, almond milk, and ice cubes until smooth.

- Enjoy a protein-packed and nutrient-rich smoothie.

Lunch: Quinoa And Chickpea Buddha Bowl
Ingredients:

- Quinoa
- Chickpeas (canned, drained, and rinsed)
- Avocado
- Cherry tomatoes
- Cucumber
- Red cabbage
- Tahini dressing

Nutritional Components (per serving):

- Protein: 14g
- Fiber: 10g
- Healthy Fats: 18g
- Vitamin C: 35% of daily value

Instructions:

- Cook quinoa according to package instructions.
- Assemble a bowl with quinoa, chickpeas, sliced avocado, cherry tomatoes, cucumber, and shredded red cabbage.

- Drizzle with tahini dressing for a satisfying Buddha Bowl.

Dinner: Shrimp And Vegetable Stir-fry With Brown Rice

Ingredients:
- Shrimp
- Mixed vegetables (broccoli, bell peppers, snap peas, carrots)
- Brown rice
- Soy sauce
- Garlic
- Ginger
- Sesame oil

Nutritional Components (per serving):
- Protein: 20g
- Fiber: 7g
- Healthy Fats: 8g
- Iron: 15% of daily value

Instructions:
- Sauté shrimp and mixed vegetables in a pan.
- Add soy sauce, minced garlic, ginger, and a drizzle of sesame oil.

- Serve over cooked brown rice for a quick and tasty stir-fry.

Snack: Greek Yogurt Parfait With Berries

Ingredients:

- Greek yogurt
- Mixed berries (strawberries, blueberries, raspberries)
- Granola

Nutritional Components (per serving):

- Protein: 10g
- Fiber: 6g
- Healthy Fats: 8g

Instructions:

- Layer Greek yogurt with mixed berries and granola for a delightful and protein-rich snack.

Dessert: Dark Chocolate-dipped Strawberries

Ingredients:

- Strawberries
- Dark chocolate (70% cocoa or higher)

Nutritional Components (per serving):
- Fiber: 5g
- Antioxidants: High

Instructions:
- Melt dark chocolate in a bowl.
- Dip strawberries into the melted chocolate and let them cool until the chocolate hardens.

Grocery List for Day 7:
Bananas, Spinach, Protein powder, Almond milk, Quinoa, Chickpeas (canned), Avocado, Cherry tomatoes, Cucumber, Red cabbage, Tahini dressing, Shrimp, Mixed vegetables (broccoli, bell peppers, snap peas, carrots), Brown rice, Soy sauce, Garlic, Ginger, Sesame oil, Greek yogurt, Mixed berries (strawberries, blueberries, raspberries), Granola, Strawberries, Dark chocolate (70% cocoa or higher).

WEEK 4 - SAVORING EXCELLENCE: A MONTH OF DASH DELIGHTS

Day 1: Tasty and Wholesome

Breakfast: Blueberry and Almond Butter Overnight Oats

Ingredients:
- Rolled oats
- Almond milk
- Blueberries
- Almond butter
- Chia seeds

Nutritional Components (per serving):
- Protein: 10g
- Fiber: 8g
- Healthy Fats: 12g
- Antioxidants: High

Instructions:
- Combine rolled oats, almond milk, blueberries, almond butter, and chia seeds in a jar.
- Refrigerate overnight for a delicious and nutrient-packed breakfast.

Lunch: Spinach and Feta Stuffed Chicken Breast

Ingredients:
- Chicken breast
- Spinach
- Feta cheese
- Olive oil
- Garlic
- Lemon
- Salt and pepper to taste

Nutritional Components (per serving):
- Protein: 25g
- Fiber: 5g
- Healthy Fats: 12g
- Vitamin C: 30% of daily value

Instructions:
- Sauté spinach, garlic, and crumbled feta cheese in olive oil until wilted.
- Slice a pocket into the chicken breast, stuff with the spinach and feta mixture, and bake until fully cooked.

Dinner: Vegetarian Chickpea Curry with Quinoa
Ingredients:
- Chickpeas (canned, drained, and rinsed)
- Coconut milk
- Tomato sauce
- Onion
- Garlic
- Ginger
- Curry powder
- Turmeric
- Cumin
- Cayenne pepper
- Quinoa

Nutritional Components (per serving):
- Protein: 18g
- Fiber: 10g
- Healthy Fats: 15g
- Iron: 20% of daily value

Instructions:
- Sauté chopped onion, garlic, and ginger in a pot.
- Add chickpeas, coconut milk, tomato sauce, curry powder, turmeric, cumin, and cayenne pepper.
- Simmer until flavors meld and serve over cooked quinoa.

Snack: Apple Slices with Peanut Butter
Ingredients:

- Apples
- Peanut butter

Nutritional Components (per serving):

- Protein: 6g
- Fiber: 4g
- Healthy Fats: 8g

Instructions:

- Slice apples and dip into peanut butter for a satisfying and nutritious snack.

Dessert: Banana and Walnut Nice Cream

Ingredients:

- Bananas (frozen)
- Walnuts

Nutritional Components (per serving):

- Protein: 8g
- Fiber: 6g
- Healthy Fats: 10g

Instructions:

- Blend frozen bananas until smooth and creamy.

- Fold in chopped walnuts for a delicious and guilt-free nice cream.

Grocery List for Day 1:
Rolled oats, Almond milk, Blueberries, Almond butter, Chia seeds, Chicken breast, Spinach, Feta cheese, Olive oil, Garlic, Lemon, Quinoa, Chickpeas (canned), Coconut milk, Tomato sauce, Onion, Ginger, Curry powder, Turmeric, Cumin, Cayenne pepper, Apples, Peanut butter, Bananas (frozen), Walnuts.

Day 2: Culmination of Delights

Breakfast: Raspberry and Almond Breakfast Parfait

Ingredients:
- Greek yogurt
- Almonds (sliced)
- Raspberries
- Honey

Nutritional Components (per serving):
- Protein: 12g
- Fiber: 6g
- Healthy Fats: 8g

Instructions:
- Layer Greek yogurt with sliced almonds and fresh raspberries.
- Drizzle with honey for a delightful and protein-rich breakfast parfait.

Lunch: Turkey and Avocado Wrap

Ingredients:
- Whole-grain wrap
- Turkey slices
- Avocado
- Lettuce
- Tomato
- Mustard

Nutritional Components (per serving):
- Protein: 15g
- Fiber: 7g
- Healthy Fats: 10g
- Vitamin C: 20% of daily value

Instructions:
- Assemble a whole-grain wrap with turkey slices, sliced avocado, lettuce, tomato, and a touch of mustard.

Dinner: Grilled Salmon with Quinoa and Asparagus

Ingredients:
- Salmon filets
- Quinoa
- Asparagus
- Lemon
- Olive oil
- Dill
- Salt and pepper to taste

Nutritional Components (per serving):
- Protein: 25g
- Fiber: 7g
- Healthy Fats: 12g
- Vitamin C: 30% of daily value

Instructions:
- Season salmon with olive oil, lemon, dill, salt, and pepper.
- Grill alongside quinoa and asparagus until fully cooked.

Snack: Greek Yogurt with Berries and Almonds

Ingredients:
- Greek yogurt
- Mixed berries (strawberries, blueberries, raspberries)

- Almonds (sliced)

Nutritional Components (per serving):
- Protein: 10g
- Fiber: 6g
- Healthy Fats: 10g

Instructions:
- Combine Greek yogurt with mixed berries and sliced almonds for a satisfying and protein-rich snack.

Dessert: Pineapple and Mint Sorbet

Ingredients:
- Pineapple (frozen)
- Fresh mint leaves

Nutritional Components (per serving):
- Fiber: 5g
- Vitamin C: 150% of daily value
- Antioxidants: High

Instructions:
- Blend frozen pineapple until smooth.
- Add fresh mint leaves and blend again for a refreshing pineapple and mint sorbet.

Grocery List for Day 2:

Greek yogurt, Almonds (sliced), Raspberries, Honey, Whole-grain wrap, Turkey slices, Avocado, Lettuce, Tomato, Mustard, Salmon filets, Quinoa, Asparagus, Lemon, Olive oil, Dill, Mixed berries (strawberries, blueberries, raspberries), Almonds (sliced), Pineapple (frozen), Fresh mint leaves

Day 3: Energizing Choices

Breakfast: Spinach and Mushroom Omelette

Ingredients:
- Eggs
- Spinach
- Mushrooms
- Feta cheese
- Olive oil
- Salt and pepper to taste

Nutritional Components (per serving):
- Protein: 14g
- Fiber: 5g
- Healthy Fats: 10g
- Iron: 20% of daily value

Instructions:

- Whisk eggs and pour into a pan.
- Add sautéed spinach, mushrooms, and crumbled feta cheese.
- Fold into an omelet and cook until set.

Lunch: Quinoa Salad with Pomegranate Seeds
Ingredients:

- Quinoa
- Pomegranate seeds
- Cucumber
- Red onion
- Mint leaves
- Feta cheese
- Balsamic vinaigrette

Nutritional Components (per serving):

- Protein: 10g
- Fiber: 8g
- Healthy Fats: 10g
- Vitamin C: 25% of daily value

Instructions:

- Cook quinoa according to package instructions.
- Mix quinoa with pomegranate seeds, diced cucumber, sliced red onion, chopped mint leaves, and crumbled feta cheese.

- Drizzle with balsamic vinaigrette for a refreshing salad.

Dinner: Baked Chicken Breast with Sweet Potato Mash

Ingredients:
- Chicken breast
- Sweet potatoes
- Olive oil
- Garlic powder
- Paprika
- Rosemary
- Salt and pepper to taste

Nutritional Components (per serving):
- Protein: 25g
- Fiber: 7g
- Healthy Fats: 10g
- Vitamin A: 300% of daily value

Instructions:
- Season chicken breast with olive oil, garlic powder, paprika, rosemary, salt, and pepper.
- Bake until fully cooked.
- Mash sweet potatoes and serve alongside the baked chicken.

Snack: Celery Sticks with Hummus

Ingredients:
- Celery sticks
- Hummus

Nutritional Components (per serving):
- Protein: 6g
- Fiber: 5g
- Healthy Fats: 8g

Instructions:
- Dip celery sticks into hummus for a crunchy and satisfying snack.

Dessert: Mango and Coconut Chia Pudding

Ingredients:
- Chia seeds
- Coconut milk
- Mango (diced)

Nutritional Components (per serving):
- Protein: 8g
- Fiber: 10g
- Healthy Fats: 12g
- Vitamin C: 60% of daily value

Instructions:
- Mix chia seeds with coconut milk and layer with diced mango.
- Refrigerate until the mixture thickens into a delightful chia pudding.

Grocery List for Day 3:
Eggs, Spinach, Mushrooms, Feta cheese, Olive oil, Quinoa, Pomegranate seeds, Cucumber, Red onion, Mint leaves, Feta cheese, Balsamic vinaigrette, Chicken breast, Sweet potatoes, Garlic powder, Paprika, Rosemary, Celery sticks, Hummus, Chia seeds, Coconut milk, Mango.

Day 4: Tasty and Wholesome

Breakfast: Banana and Walnut Pancakes

Ingredients:
- Whole-grain pancake mix
- Banana
- Walnuts
- Maple syrup

Nutritional Components (per serving):
- Protein: 8g
- Fiber: 5g
- Healthy Fats: 10g

Instructions:
- Prepare whole-grain pancake mix according to package instructions.
- Add mashed banana and chopped walnuts to the batter.
- Cook pancakes and drizzle with maple syrup.

Lunch: Lentil Soup with Spinach

Ingredients:
- Lentils
- Spinach
- Carrots
- Celery
- Onion
- Garlic
- Vegetable broth
- Cumin
- Coriander
- Turmeric
- Salt and pepper to taste

Nutritional Components (per serving):
- Protein: 12g
- Fiber: 8g
- Healthy Fats: 5g
- Iron: 15% of daily value

Instructions:

- Sauté chopped onion and garlic in a pot.
- Add lentils, diced carrots, celery, spinach, vegetable broth, cumin, coriander, turmeric, salt, and pepper.
- Simmer until lentils are tender for a hearty lentil soup.

Dinner: Grilled Veggie and Quinoa Stuffed Peppers

Ingredients:

- Quinoa
- Bell peppers (assorted colors)
- Zucchini
- Cherry tomatoes
- Red onion
- Olive oil
- Balsamic vinegar
- Fresh basil
- Feta cheese

Nutritional Components (per serving):

- Protein: 10g
- Fiber: 8g
- Healthy Fats: 8g
- Vitamin C: 150% of daily value

Instructions:
- Cook quinoa according to package instructions.
- Grill diced zucchini, cherry tomatoes, and red onion with olive oil.
- Mix grilled veggies with cooked quinoa, drizzle with balsamic vinegar, and top with fresh basil and crumbled feta cheese.

Snack: Cottage Cheese with Pineapple

Ingredients:
- Cottage cheese
- Fresh pineapple

Nutritional Components (per serving):
- Protein: 14g
- Fiber: 3g
- Healthy Fats: 5g
- Vitamin C: 80% of daily value

Instructions:
- Top cottage cheese with fresh pineapple for a delicious and protein-packed snack.

Dessert: Dark Chocolate-Covered Strawberries
Ingredients:
- Strawberries
- Dark chocolate (70% cocoa or higher)

Nutritional Components (per serving):
- Fiber: 5g
- Antioxidants: High

Instructions:
- Melt dark chocolate in a bowl.
- Dip strawberries into the melted chocolate and let them cool until the chocolate hardens.

Grocery List for Day 4:

Whole-grain pancake mix, Banana, Walnuts, Maple syrup, Lentils, Spinach, Carrots, Celery, Onion, Garlic, Vegetable broth, Cumin, Coriander, Turmeric, Bell peppers (assorted colors), Zucchini, Cherry tomatoes, Red onion, Olive oil, Balsamic vinegar, Fresh basil, Feta cheese, Cottage cheese, Fresh pineapple, Strawberries, Dark chocolate (70% cocoa or higher).

Day 5: Culmination of Delights

Breakfast: Blueberry and Almond Smoothie Bowl
Ingredients:
- Blueberries
- Almond milk
- Greek yogurt

- Almonds (sliced)
- Chia seeds

Nutritional Components (per serving):
- Protein: 12g
- Fiber: 8g
- Healthy Fats: 10g

Instructions:
- Blend blueberries, almond milk, and Greek yogurt until smooth.
- Pour into a bowl and top with sliced almonds and chia seeds for a nutritious smoothie bowl.

Lunch: Caprese Salad with Quinoa

Ingredients:
- Quinoa
- Cherry tomatoes
- Fresh mozzarella
- Basil leaves
- Balsamic glaze
- Olive oil
- Salt and pepper to taste

Nutritional Components (per serving):
- Protein: 10g
- Fiber: 8g

- Healthy Fats: 10g
- Vitamin C: 25% of daily value

Instructions:
- Cook quinoa according to package instructions.
- Assemble a salad with quinoa, halved cherry tomatoes, fresh mozzarella balls, and basil leaves.
- Drizzle with balsamic glaze and olive oil, season with salt and pepper for a refreshing Caprese Salad.

Dinner: Teriyaki Salmon with Stir-Fried Vegetables

Ingredients:
- Salmon filets
- Teriyaki sauce
- Broccoli
- Bell peppers (assorted colors)
- Snow peas
- Carrots
- Garlic
- Ginger
- Sesame oil

Nutritional Components (per serving):
- Protein: 20g
- Fiber: 8g

- Healthy Fats: 12g
- Vitamin C: 150% of daily value

Instructions:
- Marinate salmon filets in teriyaki sauce and bake until fully cooked.
- Stir-fry broccoli, bell peppers, snow peas, carrots, minced garlic, and ginger in sesame oil.
- Serve the teriyaki salmon over the stir-fried vegetables.

Snack: Apple and Almond Butter Rice Cakes

Ingredients:
- Rice cakes
- Apple
- Almond butter

Nutritional Components (per serving):
- Protein: 8g
- Fiber: 6g
- Healthy Fats: 10g

Instructions:
- Spread almond butter on rice cakes and top with sliced apple for a crunchy and satisfying snack.

Dessert: Mixed Berry Smoothie

Ingredients:
- Mixed berries (strawberries, blueberries, raspberries)
- Almond milk
- Greek yogurt
- Honey

Nutritional Components (per serving):
- Protein: 10g
- Fiber: 6g
- Healthy Fats: 8g

Instructions:
- Blend mixed berries, almond milk, Greek yogurt, and honey until smooth.
- Enjoy a refreshing mixed berry smoothie.

Grocery List for Day 5:
Blueberries, Almond milk, Greek yogurt, Almonds (sliced), Chia seeds, Quinoa, Cherry tomatoes, Fresh mozzarella, Basil leaves, Balsamic glaze, Olive oil, Salmon filets, Teriyaki sauce, Broccoli, Bell peppers (assorted colors), Snow peas, Carrots, Garlic, Ginger, Sesame oil, Rice cakes, Apple, Almond butter, Mixed berries (strawberries, blueberries, raspberries), Honey.

Day 6: Energizing Choices

Breakfast: Avocado and Tomato Toast
Ingredients:
- Whole-grain bread
- Avocado
- Cherry tomatoes
- Olive oil
- Salt and pepper to taste

Nutritional Components (per serving):
- Protein: 8g
- Fiber: 6g
- Healthy Fats: 10g
- Vitamin C: 20% of daily value

Instructions:
- Toast whole-grain bread slices.
- Spread mashed avocado on the toast and top with sliced cherry tomatoes.
- Drizzle with olive oil, sprinkle with salt and pepper for a delicious and nutritious breakfast.

Lunch: Chickpea and Vegetable Stir-Fry with Brown Rice
Ingredients:
- Chickpeas (canned, drained, and rinsed)
- Broccoli

- Carrots
- Bell peppers (assorted colors)
- Snap peas
- Soy sauce
- Garlic
- Ginger
- Brown rice

Nutritional Components (per serving):
- Protein: 15g
- Fiber: 10g
- Healthy Fats: 8g

Instructions:
- Sauté chickpeas, broccoli, carrots, bell peppers, and snap peas in a pan.
- Add soy sauce, minced garlic, and ginger.
- Serve over cooked brown rice for a quick and flavorful stir-fry.

Dinner: Turkey and Quinoa Stuffed Bell Peppers

Ingredients:
- Turkey breast (ground)
- Quinoa
- Bell peppers (assorted colors)
- Black beans (canned, drained, and rinsed)
- Corn kernels (fresh or frozen)
- Onion

- Tomato sauce
- Cumin
- Chili powder
- Paprika
- Shredded cheese

Nutritional Components (per serving):
- Protein: 20g
- Fiber: 8g
- Healthy Fats: 10g
- Vitamin C: 200% of daily value

Instructions:
- Cook quinoa according to package instructions.
- Sauté ground turkey, onion, and add black beans, corn kernels, tomato sauce, cumin, chili powder, and paprika.
- Cut bell peppers in half, stuff with the quinoa and turkey mixture, and top with shredded cheese. Bake until the cheese is melted and bubbly.

Snack: Greek Yogurt with Berries and Almonds
Ingredients:
- Greek yogurt
- Mixed berries (strawberries, blueberries, raspberries)
- Almonds (sliced)

Nutritional Components (per serving):
- Protein: 12g
- Fiber: 6g
- Healthy Fats: 10g

Instructions:
- Combine Greek yogurt with mixed berries and sliced almonds for a satisfying and protein-rich snack.

Dessert: Chocolate-Dipped Banana Slices

Ingredients:
- Bananas
- Dark chocolate (70% cocoa or higher)

Nutritional Components (per serving):
- Fiber: 5g
- Antioxidants: High

Instructions:
- Slice bananas and dip them into melted dark chocolate.
- Let them cool until the chocolate hardens for a sweet and satisfying dessert.

Grocery List for Day 6:

Whole-grain bread, Avocado, Cherry tomatoes, Olive oil, Chickpeas (canned), Broccoli, Carrots, Bell peppers (assorted colors), Snap peas, Soy sauce, Garlic, Ginger, Brown rice, Turkey breast (ground), Quinoa, Black beans (canned), Corn kernels (fresh or frozen), Onion, Tomato sauce, Cumin, Chili powder, Paprika, Shredded cheese, Greek yogurt, Mixed berries (strawberries, blueberries, raspberries), Almonds (sliced), Bananas, Dark chocolate (70% cocoa or higher).

Day 7: Culmination of Delights

Breakfast: Spinach and Feta Omelette

Ingredients:
- Eggs
- Spinach
- Feta cheese
- Olive oil
- Salt and pepper to taste

Nutritional Components (per serving):
- Protein: 14g
- Fiber: 5g
- Healthy Fats: 10g
- Iron: 20% of daily value

Instructions:
- Whisk eggs and pour into a pan.
- Add sautéed spinach and crumbled feta cheese.
- Fold into an omelet and cook until set.

Lunch: Quinoa Salad with Avocado and Black Beans

Ingredients:
- Quinoa
- Avocado
- Black beans (canned, drained, and rinsed)
- Corn kernels (fresh or frozen)
- Red onion
- Cilantro
- Lime
- Olive oil
- Salt and pepper to taste

Nutritional Components (per serving):
- Protein: 12g
- Fiber: 10g
- Healthy Fats: 15g
- Vitamin C: 20% of daily value

Instructions:
- Cook quinoa according to package instructions.
- Mix quinoa with diced avocado, black beans, corn kernels, diced red onion, chopped cilantro, lime juice, olive oil, salt, and pepper for a refreshing salad.

Dinner: Grilled Chicken Breast with Sweet Potato Wedges

Ingredients:
- Chicken breast
- Sweet potatoes
- Olive oil
- Garlic powder
- Paprika
- Rosemary
- Salt and pepper to taste

Nutritional Components (per serving):
- Protein: 25g
- Fiber: 7g
- Healthy Fats: 10g
- Vitamin A: 300% of daily value

Instructions:
- Season chicken breast with olive oil, garlic powder, paprika, rosemary, salt, and pepper.

- Grill until fully cooked.
- Cut sweet potatoes into wedges, toss with olive oil, and bake until crispy.

Snack: Hummus and Vegetable Sticks
Ingredients:
- Hummus
- Carrot sticks
- Cucumber slices
- Bell pepper strips

Nutritional Components (per serving):
- Protein: 6g
- Fiber: 5g
- Healthy Fats: 8g

Instructions:
- Dip carrot sticks, cucumber slices, and bell pepper strips into hummus for a crunchy and satisfying snack.

Dessert: Mixed Berry Parfait

Ingredients:
- Greek yogurt
- Mixed berries (strawberries, blueberries, raspberries)
- Granola

Nutritional Components (per serving):
- Protein: 10g
- Fiber: 6g
- Healthy Fats: 8g

Instructions:
- Layer Greek yogurt with mixed berries and granola for a delightful and protein-rich dessert.

Grocery List for Day 7:

Eggs, Spinach, Feta cheese, Olive oil, Quinoa, Avocado, Black beans (canned), Corn kernels (fresh or frozen), Red onion, Cilantro, Lime, Sweet potatoes, Garlic powder, Paprika, Rosemary, Chicken breast, Carrot sticks, Cucumber, Bell peppers, Hummus, Greek yogurt, Mixed berries (strawberries, blueberries, raspberries), Granola.

WEEK 5- DASH DIET ADVENTURES: EXPLORING WHIRLWINDS OF FLAVOR

Day 1: Energizing Choices

Breakfast: Berry and Almond Overnight Oats

Ingredients:
- Rolled oats
- Almond milk
- Mixed berries (strawberries, blueberries, raspberries)
- Almonds (sliced)
- Honey

Nutritional Components (per serving):
- Protein: 10g
- Fiber: 8g
- Healthy Fats: 10g

Instructions:
- Mix rolled oats with almond milk and refrigerate overnight.
- In the morning, top with mixed berries, sliced almonds, and a drizzle of honey for a quick and nutritious breakfast.

Lunch: Mediterranean Chickpea Salad

Ingredients:
- Chickpeas (canned, drained, and rinsed)
- Cucumber
- Cherry tomatoes
- Kalamata olives
- Red onion
- Feta cheese
- Olive oil
- Lemon juice
- Oregano
- Salt and pepper to taste

Nutritional Components (per serving):
- Protein: 12g
- Fiber: 8g
- Healthy Fats: 15g

Instructions:
- Combine chickpeas, diced cucumber, halved cherry tomatoes, sliced Kalamata olives, diced red onion, and crumbled feta cheese in a bowl.
- Drizzle with olive oil and lemon juice, sprinkle with oregano, salt, and pepper for a refreshing Mediterranean salad.

Dinner: Teriyaki Tofu Stir-Fry with Brown Rice

Ingredients:
- Firm tofu
- Broccoli
- Bell peppers (assorted colors)
- Carrots
- Snap peas
- Teriyaki sauce
- Garlic
- Ginger
- Brown rice

Nutritional Components (per serving):
- Protein: 15g
- Fiber: 10g
- Healthy Fats: 8g

Instructions:
- Press and cube firm tofu.
- Stir-fry tofu, broccoli, bell peppers, carrots, and snap peas in teriyaki sauce, minced garlic, and ginger.
- Serve over cooked brown rice for a delicious and plant-based stir-fry.

Snack: Apple and Almond Butter

Ingredients:

- Apple
- Almond butter

Nutritional Components (per serving):

- Protein: 6g
- Fiber: 4g
- Healthy Fats: 8g

Instructions:

- Slice the apple and dip it into almond butter for a satisfying and nutritious snack.

Dessert: Mango and Coconut Chia Pudding

Ingredients:

- Chia seeds
- Coconut milk
- Mango (diced)

Nutritional Components (per serving):

- Protein: 8g
- Fiber: 10g
- Healthy Fats: 12g
- Vitamin C: 60% of daily value

Instructions:
- Mix chia seeds with coconut milk and layer with diced mango.
- Refrigerate until the mixture thickens into a delightful chia pudding.

Grocery List for Day 1:

Rolled oats, Almond milk, Mixed berries (strawberries, blueberries, raspberries), Almonds (sliced), Honey, Chickpeas (canned), Cucumber, Cherry tomatoes, Kalamata olives, Red onion, Feta cheese, Olive oil, Lemon, Oregano, Salt, Pepper, Firm tofu, Broccoli, Bell peppers (assorted colors), Carrots, Snap peas, Teriyaki sauce, Garlic, Ginger, Brown rice, Apple, Almond butter, Chia seeds, Coconut milk, Mango.

Day 2: Culmination of Delights

Breakfast: Peanut Butter and Banana Smoothie

Ingredients:
- Banana
- Peanut butter
- Greek yogurt
- Almond milk
- Ice cubes

Nutritional Components (per serving):
- Protein: 12g
- Fiber: 6g
- Healthy Fats: 10g

Instructions:
- Blend banana, peanut butter, Greek yogurt, almond milk, and ice cubes until smooth.
- Enjoy a creamy and protein-packed smoothie.

Lunch: Quinoa Bowl with Roasted Vegetables

Ingredients:
- Quinoa
- Sweet potatoes
- Brussels sprouts
- Red onion
- Olive oil
- Balsamic vinegar
- Maple syrup
- Salt and pepper to taste

Nutritional Components (per serving):
- Protein: 10g
- Fiber: 8g
- Healthy Fats: 10g
- Vitamin A: 200% of daily value

Instructions:

- Cook quinoa according to package instructions.
- Roast sweet potatoes, Brussels sprouts, and red onion with olive oil, balsamic vinegar, maple syrup, salt, and pepper.
- Serve over quinoa for a nutritious and flavorful bowl.

Dinner: Lemon Herb Grilled Shrimp with Quinoa Salad

Ingredients:

- Shrimp
- Lemon
- Olive oil
- Garlic
- Fresh parsley
- Quinoa
- Cucumber
- Cherry tomatoes
- Red bell pepper
- Feta cheese
- Red wine vinegar
- Salt and pepper to taste

Nutritional Components (per serving):
- Protein: 20g
- Fiber: 8g
- Healthy Fats: 12g
- Vitamin C: 80% of daily value

Instructions:
- Marinate shrimp in lemon juice, olive oil, minced garlic, and chopped fresh parsley.
- Grill shrimp until cooked through.
- Mix quinoa with diced cucumber, halved cherry tomatoes, diced red bell pepper, crumbled feta cheese, red wine vinegar, salt, and pepper. Serve the grilled shrimp over the quinoa salad.

Snack: Celery Sticks with Hummus

Ingredients:
- Celery sticks
- Hummus

Nutritional Components (per serving):
- Protein: 6g
- Fiber: 5g
- Healthy Fats: 8g

Instructions:
- Dip celery sticks into hummus for a crunchy and satisfying snack.

Dessert: Dark Chocolate-Covered Strawberries

Ingredients:
- Strawberries
- Dark chocolate (70% cocoa or higher)

Nutritional Components (per serving):
- Fiber: 5g
- Antioxidants: High

Instructions:
- Melt dark chocolate in a bowl.
- Dip strawberries into the melted chocolate and let them cool until the chocolate hardens.

Grocery List for Day 2:
Banana, Peanut butter, Greek yogurt, Almond milk, Ice cubes, Quinoa, Sweet potatoes, Brussels sprouts, Red onion, Olive oil, Balsamic vinegar, Maple syrup, Shrimp, Lemon, Garlic, Fresh parsley, Cucumber, Cherry tomatoes, Red bell pepper, Feta cheese, Red wine vinegar, Celery sticks, Hummus, Strawberries, Dark chocolate (70% cocoa or higher).

Day 3: Energizing Choices

Breakfast: Greek Yogurt Parfait with Berries and Granola

Ingredients:
- Greek yogurt
- Mixed berries (strawberries, blueberries, raspberries)
- Granola

Nutritional Components (per serving):
- Protein: 12g
- Fiber: 6g
- Healthy Fats: 8g

Instructions:
- Layer Greek yogurt with mixed berries and granola for a delightful and protein-rich parfait.

Lunch: Spinach and Feta Stuffed Chicken Breast

Ingredients:
- Chicken breast
- Spinach
- Feta cheese
- Olive oil

- Garlic
- Lemon
- Salt and pepper to taste

Nutritional Components (per serving):
- Protein: 25g
- Fiber: 5g
- Healthy Fats: 10g
- Iron: 15% of daily value

Instructions:
- Sauté spinach with garlic and olive oil until wilted.
- Butterfly the chicken breast, stuff with sautéed spinach and feta cheese.
- Grill or bake until fully cooked. Squeeze fresh lemon juice over the top before serving.

Dinner: Quinoa and Black Bean Stuffed Bell Peppers

Ingredients:
- Quinoa
- Black beans (canned, drained, and rinsed)
- Bell peppers (assorted colors)
- Corn kernels (fresh or frozen)
- Onion
- Tomato sauce

- Cumin
- Chili powder
- Paprika
- Shredded cheese

Nutritional Components (per serving):
- Protein: 15g
- Fiber: 10g
- Healthy Fats: 8g
- Vitamin C: 150% of daily value

Instructions:
- Cook quinoa according to package instructions.
- Mix quinoa with black beans, corn kernels, diced onion, tomato sauce, cumin, chili powder, and paprika.
- Cut bell peppers in half, stuff with the quinoa and black bean mixture, and top with shredded cheese. Bake until the cheese is melted and bubbly.

Snack: Cottage Cheese with Pineapple

Ingredients:
- Cottage cheese
- Fresh pineapple

Nutritional Components (per serving):
- Protein: 14g
- Fiber: 3g
- Healthy Fats: 5g
- Vitamin C: 80% of daily value

Instructions:
- Top cottage cheese with fresh pineapple for a protein-packed and refreshing snack.

Dessert: Dark Chocolate-Covered Almonds

Ingredients:
- Almonds
- Dark chocolate (70% cocoa or higher)

Nutritional Components (per serving):
- Protein: 6g
- Fiber: 4g
- Healthy Fats: 10g

Instructions:
- Melt dark chocolate and dip almonds into the melted chocolate.
- Let them cool until the chocolate hardens for a sweet and satisfying dessert.

Grocery List for Day 3:

Greek yogurt, Mixed berries (strawberries, blueberries, raspberries), Granola, Chicken breast, Spinach, Feta cheese, Olive oil, Garlic, Lemon, Quinoa, Black beans (canned), Bell peppers (assorted colors), Corn kernels (fresh or frozen), Onion, Tomato sauce, Cumin, Chili powder, Paprika, Shredded cheese, Cottage cheese, Fresh pineapple, Almonds, Dark chocolate (70% cocoa or higher).

Day 4: Culmination of Delights

Breakfast: Blueberry and Almond Smoothie Bowl

Ingredients:
- Blueberries
- Almond milk
- Greek yogurt
- Almonds (sliced)
- Chia seeds

Nutritional Components (per serving):
- Protein: 12g
- Fiber: 8g
- Healthy Fats: 10g

Instructions:

- Blend blueberries, almond milk, and Greek yogurt until smooth.
- Pour into a bowl and top with sliced almonds and chia seeds for a nutritious smoothie bowl.

Lunch: Lentil Soup with Spinach

Ingredients:

- Lentils
- Spinach
- Carrots
- Celery
- Onion
- Garlic
- Vegetable broth
- Cumin
- Coriander
- Turmeric
- Salt and pepper to taste

Nutritional Components (per serving):

- Protein: 12g
- Fiber: 8g
- Healthy Fats: 5g
- Iron: 15% of daily value

Instructions:
- Sauté chopped onion and garlic in a pot.
- Add lentils, diced carrots, celery, spinach, vegetable broth, cumin, coriander, turmeric, salt, and pepper.
- Simmer until lentils are tender for a hearty lentil soup.

Dinner: Grilled Veggie and Quinoa Stuffed Peppers

Ingredients:
- Quinoa
- Bell peppers (assorted colors)
- Zucchini
- Cherry tomatoes
- Red onion
- Olive oil
- Balsamic vinegar
- Fresh basil
- Feta cheese

Nutritional Components (per serving):
- Protein: 10g
- Fiber: 8g
- Healthy Fats: 8g
- Vitamin C: 150% of daily value

Instructions:

- Cook quinoa according to package instructions.
- Grill diced zucchini, cherry tomatoes, and red onion with olive oil.
- Mix grilled veggies with cooked quinoa, fresh basil, and crumbled feta cheese.
- Stuff bell peppers with the quinoa and veggie mixture.
- Drizzle with balsamic vinegar before serving.

Snack: Banana and Walnut Energy Bites

Ingredients:

- Bananas
- Walnuts
- Rolled oats
- Honey
- Cinnamon

Nutritional Components (per serving):

- Protein: 6g
- Fiber: 4g
- Healthy Fats: 8g

Instructions:

- Mash bananas and mix with crushed walnuts, rolled oats, honey, and cinnamon.

- Form into small energy bites and refrigerate.

Dessert: Berry and Yogurt Popsicles

Ingredients:
- Mixed berries (strawberries, blueberries, raspberries)
- Greek yogurt
- Honey

Nutritional Components (per serving):
- Protein: 8g
- Fiber: 4g
- Healthy Fats: 6g

Instructions:
- Blend mixed berries with Greek yogurt and honey.
- Pour into popsicle molds and freeze until solid.

Grocery List for Day 4:
Blueberries, Almond milk, Greek yogurt, Almonds (sliced), Chia seeds, Lentils, Spinach, Carrots, Celery, Onion, Garlic, Vegetable broth, Cumin, Coriander, Turmeric, Salt, Pepper, Quinoa, Bell peppers (assorted colors), Zucchini, Cherry tomatoes, Red onion, Olive oil, Balsamic vinegar, Fresh basil, Feta cheese, Bananas, Walnuts, Rolled

oats, Honey, Cinnamon, Mixed berries (strawberries, blueberries, raspberries).

Day 5: Energizing Choices

Breakfast: Mango and Pineapple Smoothie Bowl

Ingredients:
- Mango
- Pineapple
- Coconut milk
- Greek yogurt
- Granola
- Shredded coconut

Nutritional Components (per serving):
- Protein: 10g
- Fiber: 6g
- Healthy Fats: 8g

Instructions:
- Blend mango, pineapple, coconut milk, and Greek yogurt until smooth.
- Pour into a bowl and top with granola and shredded coconut for a tropical smoothie bowl.

Lunch: Caprese Salad with Balsamic Glaze

Ingredients:
- Tomatoes
- Fresh mozzarella
- Fresh basil
- Olive oil
- Balsamic glaze
- Salt and pepper to taste

Nutritional Components (per serving):
- Protein: 12g
- Healthy Fats: 15g
- Vitamin C: 30% of daily value

Instructions:
- Slice tomatoes and fresh mozzarella.
- Arrange on a plate with fresh basil leaves.
- Drizzle with olive oil and balsamic glaze.
- Sprinkle it with salt and pepper for a refreshing Caprese salad.

Dinner: Teriyaki Salmon with Quinoa and Broccoli

Ingredients:
- Salmon filets
- Teriyaki sauce
- Quinoa

- Broccoli
- Sesame seeds
- Green onions

Nutritional Components (per serving):
- Protein: 20g
- Fiber: 8g
- Healthy Fats: 10g

Instructions:
- Marinate salmon filets in teriyaki sauce.
- Bake or grill until salmon is cooked through.
- Serve over cooked quinoa and steamed broccoli.
- Garnish with sesame seeds and chopped green onions.

Snack: Greek Yogurt with Honey and Walnuts

Ingredients:
- Greek yogurt
- Honey
- Walnuts

Nutritional Components (per serving):
- Protein: 14g
- Healthy Fats: 10g

Instructions:
- Top Greek yogurt with a drizzle of honey and crushed walnuts for a protein-packed snack.

Dessert: Dark Chocolate-Dipped Mango Slices

Ingredients:
- Mango
- Dark chocolate (70% cocoa or higher)

Nutritional Components (per serving):
- Fiber: 5g
- Antioxidants: High

Instructions:
- Slice mango and dip into melted dark chocolate.
- Let them cool until the chocolate hardens for a sweet and satisfying dessert.

Grocery List for Day 5:
Mango, Pineapple, Coconut milk, Greek yogurt, Granola, Shredded coconut, Tomatoes, Fresh mozzarella, Fresh basil, Olive oil, Balsamic glaze, Salmon filets, Teriyaki sauce, Quinoa, Broccoli, Sesame seeds, Green onions, Greek yogurt, Honey, Walnuts, Dark chocolate (70% cocoa or higher).

Day 6: Culmination of Delights

Breakfast: Avocado and Tomato Toast with Poached Egg

Ingredients:
- Whole-grain bread
- Avocado
- Cherry tomatoes
- Eggs
- Olive oil
- Salt and pepper to taste

Nutritional Components (per serving):
- Protein: 12g
- Fiber: 6g
- Healthy Fats: 15g

Instructions:
- Toast whole-grain bread.
- Spread mashed avocado on the toast and top with sliced cherry tomatoes.
- Poach eggs and place them on top.
- Drizzle with olive oil and sprinkle with salt and pepper for a satisfying breakfast.

Lunch: Quinoa and Chickpea Salad with Lemon Vinaigrette

Ingredients:
- Quinoa
- Chickpeas (canned, drained, and rinsed)
- Cucumber
- Red bell pepper
- Red onion
- Feta cheese
- Kalamata olives
- Olive oil
- Lemon
- Dijon mustard
- Honey
- Salt and pepper to taste

Nutritional Components (per serving):
- Protein: 14g
- Fiber: 10g
- Healthy Fats: 12g

Instructions:
- Cook quinoa according to package instructions.
- Combine quinoa with chickpeas, diced cucumber, diced red bell pepper, diced red onion, crumbled feta cheese, and sliced Kalamata olives.

- In a separate bowl, whisk together olive oil, lemon juice, Dijon mustard, honey, salt, and pepper to make the lemon vinaigrette.
- Pour the vinaigrette over the salad and toss gently.

Dinner: Grilled Chicken Caesar Salad

Ingredients:
- Chicken breast
- Romaine lettuce
- Cherry tomatoes
- Croutons
- Parmesan cheese
- Caesar dressing

Nutritional Components (per serving):
- Protein: 25g
- Fiber: 6g
- Healthy Fats: 12g

Instructions:
- Season chicken breast with salt and pepper.
- Grill until fully cooked.
- Slice grilled chicken and arrange on a bed of chopped Romaine lettuce.
- Add halved cherry tomatoes, croutons, and shaved Parmesan cheese.

- Drizzle with Caesar dressing for a classic and protein-packed salad.

Snack: Apple Slices with Almond Butter

Ingredients:
- Apple
- Almond butter

Nutritional Components (per serving):
- Protein: 6g
- Fiber: 4g
- Healthy Fats: 8g

Instructions:
- Slice the apple and dip it into almond butter for a quick and satisfying snack.

Dessert: Mixed Berry Yogurt Parfait

Ingredients:
- Greek yogurt
- Mixed berries (strawberries, blueberries, raspberries)
- Honey
- Granola

Nutritional Components (per serving):
- Protein: 12g
- Fiber: 6g
- Healthy Fats: 8g

Instructions:
- Layer Greek yogurt with mixed berries, a drizzle of honey, and granola for a delightful and protein-rich dessert.

Grocery List for Day 6:

Whole-grain bread, Avocado, Cherry tomatoes, Eggs, Olive oil, Salt, Pepper, Quinoa, Chickpeas (canned), Cucumber, Red bell pepper, Red onion, Feta cheese, Kalamata olives, Lemon, Dijon mustard, Honey, Romaine lettuce, Croutons, Parmesan cheese, Caesar dressing, Apple, Almond butter, Mixed berries (strawberries, blueberries, raspberries), Honey, Granola.

Day 7: Culmination of Delights

Breakfast: Spinach and Mushroom Omelette

Ingredients:
- Eggs
- Spinach
- Mushrooms

- Feta cheese
- Olive oil
- Salt and pepper to taste

Nutritional Components (per serving):
- Protein: 15g
- Fiber: 4g
- Healthy Fats: 10g

Instructions:
- Sauté spinach and mushrooms in olive oil until tender.
- Whisk eggs and pour them over the sautéed vegetables.
- Cook until the eggs are set, fold in half, and sprinkle with crumbled feta cheese.
- Season with salt and pepper for a nutritious and protein-packed omelet..

Lunch: Mediterranean Quinoa Bowl

Ingredients:
- Quinoa
- Chickpeas (canned, drained, and rinsed)
- Cherry tomatoes
- Cucumber
- Red onion
- Kalamata olives

- Feta cheese
- Olive oil
- Lemon juice
- Oregano
- Salt and pepper to taste

Nutritional Components (per serving):
- Protein: 14g
- Fiber: 10g
- Healthy Fats: 12g

Instructions:
- Cook quinoa according to package instructions.
- Combine quinoa with chickpeas, halved cherry tomatoes, diced cucumber, diced red onion, sliced Kalamata olives, and crumbled feta cheese.
- Drizzle with olive oil, lemon juice, sprinkle with oregano, salt, and pepper for a refreshing Mediterranean quinoa bowl.

Dinner: Stir-Fried Tofu with Broccoli and Brown Rice

Ingredients:
- Firm tofu
- Broccoli
- Soy sauce

- Sesame oil
- Garlic
- Ginger
- Brown rice

Nutritional Components (per serving):
- Protein: 20g
- Fiber: 8g
- Healthy Fats: 10g

Instructions:
- Press and cube firm tofu.
- Stir-fry tofu and broccoli in a mixture of soy sauce, sesame oil, minced garlic, and ginger.
- Serve over cooked brown rice for a quick and nutritious stir-fry.

Snack: Greek Yogurt and Berry Smoothie

Ingredients:
- Greek yogurt
- Mixed berries (strawberries, blueberries, raspberries)
- Honey
- Ice cubes

Nutritional Components (per serving):
- Protein: 12g
- Fiber: 6g

- Healthy Fats: 8g

Instructions:
- Blend Greek yogurt, mixed berries, honey, and ice cubes until smooth.
- Enjoy a creamy and protein-packed smoothie as a refreshing snack.

Dessert: Dark Chocolate-Covered Banana Slices

Ingredients:
- Banana
- Dark chocolate (70% cocoa or higher)

Nutritional Components (per serving):
- Fiber: 4g
- Antioxidants: High

Instructions:
- Slice banana and dip into melted dark chocolate.
- Let them cool until the chocolate hardens for a sweet and satisfying dessert.

Grocery List for Day 7:
Eggs, Spinach, Mushrooms, Feta cheese, Olive oil, Salt, Pepper, Quinoa, Chickpeas (canned), Cherry tomatoes, Cucumber, Red onion, Kalamata olives, Feta cheese, Olive oil, Lemon, Oregano, Salt,

Pepper, Firm tofu, Broccoli, Soy sauce, Sesame oil, Garlic, Ginger, Brown rice, Greek yogurt, Mixed berries (strawberries, blueberries, raspberries), Honey, Ice cubes, Banana, Dark chocolate (70% cocoa or higher).

WEEK 6: FLAVORS IN FULL BLOOM: NOURISHING BODY AND SOUL WITH DASH DELICACIES

Day 1: Energizing Beginnings

Breakfast: Banana and Almond Butter Smoothie Bowl

Ingredients:
- Banana
- Almond butter
- Almond milk
- Greek yogurt
- Granola
- Chia seeds

Nutritional Components (per serving):
- Protein: 12g
- Fiber: 8g
- Healthy Fats: 10g

Instructions:
- Blend banana, almond butter, almond milk, and Greek yogurt until smooth.
- Pour into a bowl and top with granola and chia seeds for a nutritious and satisfying smoothie bowl.

Lunch: Quinoa and Black Bean Burrito Bowl

Ingredients:
- Quinoa
- Black beans (canned, drained, and rinsed)
- Corn kernels
- Avocado
- Cherry tomatoes
- Lime
- Cilantro
- Salsa

Nutritional Components (per serving):
- Protein: 14g
- Fiber: 10g
- Healthy Fats: 10g
- Vitamin C: 20% of daily value

Instructions:
- Cook quinoa according to package instructions.
- Assemble a bowl with quinoa, black beans, corn kernels, diced avocado, halved cherry tomatoes, a squeeze of lime juice, and fresh cilantro.
- Top with salsa for a delicious and satisfying burrito bowl.

Dinner: Baked Lemon Herb Chicken with Roasted Vegetables

Ingredients:
- Chicken thighs
- Lemon
- Garlic
- Thyme
- Rosemary
- Olive oil
- Sweet potatoes
- Brussels sprouts
- Salt and pepper to taste

Nutritional Components (per serving):
- Protein: 25g
- Fiber: 8g
- Healthy Fats: 12g
- Vitamin A: 150% of daily value

Instructions:
- Marinate chicken thighs in a mixture of lemon juice, minced garlic, thyme, rosemary, and olive oil.
- Bake until chicken is cooked through.
- Roast sweet potatoes and Brussels sprouts with olive oil, salt, and pepper.

- Serve the chicken over a bed of roasted vegetables for a flavorful and nutritious dinner.

Snack: Cottage Cheese and Pineapple

Ingredients:
- Cottage cheese
- Fresh pineapple

Nutritional Components (per serving):
- Protein: 14g
- Vitamin C: 80% of daily value

Instructions:
- Combine cottage cheese with fresh pineapple for a protein-packed and refreshing snack.

Dessert: Mixed Berry Parfait with Greek Yogurt

Ingredients:
- Greek yogurt
- Mixed berries (strawberries, blueberries, raspberries)
- Honey
- Granola

Nutritional Components (per serving):
- Protein: 12g
- Fiber: 6g
- Healthy Fats: 8g

Instructions:
- Layer Greek yogurt with mixed berries, a drizzle of honey, and granola for a delightful and protein-rich dessert.

Grocery List for Day 1:

Banana, Almond butter, Almond milk, Greek yogurt, Granola, Chia seeds, Quinoa, Black beans (canned), Corn kernels, Avocado, Cherry tomatoes, Lime, Cilantro, Salsa, Chicken thighs, Lemon, Garlic, Thyme, Rosemary, Olive oil, Sweet potatoes, Brussels sprouts, Cottage cheese, Fresh pineapple, Mixed berries (strawberries, blueberries, raspberries), Honey.

Day 2: Fusion Flavors

Breakfast: Mango and Coconut Chia Pudding

Ingredients:
- Chia seeds
- Coconut milk
- Mango

- Shredded coconut

Nutritional Components (per serving):
- Protein: 8g
- Fiber: 10g
- Healthy Fats: 12g

Instructions:
- Mix chia seeds with coconut milk and let it sit in the refrigerator overnight.
- Top with diced mango and shredded coconut for a tropical and nutrient-rich breakfast.

Lunch: Spinach and Feta Stuffed Turkey Burger

Ingredients:
- Ground turkey
- Spinach
- Feta cheese
- Whole-grain bun
- Tomato
- Red onion
- Lettuce

Nutritional Components (per serving):
- Protein: 20g
- Fiber: 6g
- Healthy Fats: 8g

Instructions:

- Mix ground turkey with chopped spinach and crumbled feta cheese.
- Shape into a burger patty and grill until fully cooked.
- Serve on a whole-grain bun with sliced tomato, red onion, and lettuce.

Dinner: Teriyaki Tofu Stir-Fry with Brown Rice

Ingredients:

- Firm tofu
- Broccoli
- Carrots
- Snap peas
- Bell peppers (assorted colors)
- Brown rice
- Teriyaki sauce
- Sesame oil
- Ginger
- Garlic
- Green onions

Nutritional Components (per serving):

- Protein: 18g
- Fiber: 10g
- Healthy Fats: 8g

Instructions:

- Press and cube firm tofu.
- Stir-fry tofu, broccoli, carrots, snap peas, and bell peppers in a mixture of teriyaki sauce, sesame oil, minced ginger, and garlic.
- Serve over cooked brown rice and garnish with chopped green onions for a flavorful and satisfying stir-fry.

Snack: Apple and Almond Butter Rice Cakes

Ingredients:

- Rice cakes
- Apple
- Almond butter

Nutritional Components (per serving):

- Protein: 6g
- Fiber: 4g
- Healthy Fats: 8g

Instructions:

- Spread almond butter on rice cakes and top with sliced apple for a crunchy and satisfying snack.

Dessert: Dark Chocolate-Covered Strawberries

Ingredients:
- Strawberries
- Dark chocolate (70% cocoa or higher)

Nutritional Components (per serving):
- Fiber: 4g
- Antioxidants: High

Instructions:
- Dip strawberries into melted dark chocolate.
- Let them cool until the chocolate hardens for a sweet and guilt-free dessert.

Grocery List for Day 2:
Chia seeds, Coconut milk, Mango, Shredded coconut, Ground turkey, Spinach, Feta cheese, Whole-grain bun, Tomato, Red onion, Lettuce, Firm tofu, Broccoli, Carrots, Snap peas, Bell peppers (assorted colors), Brown rice, Teriyaki sauce, Sesame oil, Ginger, Garlic, Green onions, Rice cakes, Apple, Almond butter, Strawberries, Dark chocolate (70% cocoa or higher).

Day 3: Mediterranean Delights

Breakfast: Greek Yogurt Parfait with Pistachios

Ingredients:
- Greek yogurt
- Mixed berries (strawberries, blueberries, raspberries)
- Honey
- Pistachios (chopped)

Nutritional Components (per serving):
- Protein: 14g
- Fiber: 6g
- Healthy Fats: 10g

Instructions:
- Layer Greek yogurt with mixed berries, a drizzle of honey, and chopped pistachios for a Mediterranean-inspired parfait.

Lunch: Hummus and Veggie Wrap

Ingredients:
- Whole-grain wrap
- Hummus
- Cucumber
- Cherry tomatoes
- Red bell pepper

- Red onion
- Lettuce

Nutritional Components (per serving):
- Protein: 10g
- Fiber: 8g
- Healthy Fats: 8g
- Vitamin C: 80% of daily value

Instructions:
- Spread hummus on a whole-grain wrap.
- Fill with sliced cucumber, halved cherry tomatoes, diced red bell pepper, thinly sliced red onion, and lettuce.
- Roll up the wrap for a tasty and nutrient-packed lunch.

Dinner: Lemon Garlic Shrimp with Quinoa

Ingredients:
- Shrimp
- Quinoa
- Lemon
- Garlic
- Olive oil
- Fresh parsley
- Salt and pepper to taste

Nutritional Components (per serving):
- Protein: 20g
- Fiber: 6g
- Healthy Fats: 8g

Instructions:
- Marinate shrimp in a mixture of minced garlic, olive oil, lemon juice, chopped fresh parsley, salt, and pepper.
- Cook shrimp until they turn pink and opaque.
- Serve over cooked quinoa for a light and flavorful dinner.

Snack: Cottage Cheese and Pineapple Skewers

Ingredients:
- Cottage cheese
- Fresh pineapple
- Skewers

Nutritional Components (per serving):
- Protein: 14g
- Vitamin C: 80% of daily value

Instructions:
- Thread chunks of fresh pineapple and spoonfuls of cottage cheese onto skewers for a protein-packed and refreshing snack.

Dessert: Berry and Almond Butter Smoothie

Ingredients:
- Mixed berries (strawberries, blueberries, raspberries)
- Almond butter
- Almond milk
- Ice cubes

Nutritional Components (per serving):
- Protein: 10g
- Fiber: 8g
- Healthy Fats: 10g

Instructions:
- Blend mixed berries, almond butter, almond milk, and ice cubes until smooth.
- Sip on this delightful berry smoothie for a sweet ending to your day.

Grocery List for Day 3:
Greek yogurt, Mixed berries (strawberries, blueberries, raspberries), Honey, Pistachios (chopped), Whole-grain wrap, Hummus, Cucumber, Cherry tomatoes, Red bell pepper, Red onion, Lettuce, Shrimp, Quinoa, Lemon, Garlic, Olive oil, Fresh parsley, Salt, Pepper, Cottage cheese, Fresh

pineapple, Skewers, Almond butter, Almond milk, Ice cubes.

Day 4: Vibrant Fusion

Breakfast: Avocado and Tomato Breakfast Burrito

Ingredients:
- Whole-grain tortilla
- Eggs
- Avocado
- Cherry tomatoes
- Salsa
- Cilantro
- Salt and pepper to taste

Nutritional Components (per serving):
- Protein: 12g
- Fiber: 8g
- Healthy Fats: 15g

Instructions:
- Scramble eggs and fill a whole-grain tortilla.
- Top with sliced avocado, halved cherry tomatoes, salsa, and fresh cilantro.
- Season with salt and pepper for a nutritious breakfast burrito.

Lunch: Caprese Quinoa Salad

Ingredients:
- Quinoa
- Cherry tomatoes
- Fresh mozzarella
- Fresh basil
- Balsamic glaze
- Olive oil
- Salt and pepper to taste

Nutritional Components (per serving):
- Protein: 14g
- Healthy Fats: 15g
- Vitamin C: 30% of daily value

Instructions:
- Cook quinoa according to package instructions.
- Mix cooked quinoa with halved cherry tomatoes, diced fresh mozzarella, and fresh basil.
- Drizzle with balsamic glaze and olive oil.
- Season with salt and pepper for a refreshing Caprese quinoa salad.

Dinner: Teriyaki Salmon Poke Bowl
Ingredients:
- Salmon filets
- Teriyaki sauce
- Brown rice
- Avocado
- Cucumber
- Edamame
- Seaweed sheets
- Sesame seeds
- Green onions

Nutritional Components (per serving):
- Protein: 20g
- Fiber: 8g
- Healthy Fats: 12g

Instructions:
- Marinate salmon filets in teriyaki sauce and grill until cooked through.
- Serve grilled salmon over a bowl of cooked brown rice.
- Top with sliced avocado, cucumber, edamame, shredded seaweed sheets, sesame seeds, and chopped green onions for a delicious poke bowl.

Snack: Nut and Berry Trail Mix

Ingredients:
- Almonds
- Walnuts
- Dried cranberries
- Dark chocolate chips

Nutritional Components (per serving):
- Protein: 8g
- Fiber: 6g
- Healthy Fats: 12g

Instructions:
- Mix almonds, walnuts, dried cranberries, and dark chocolate chips for a crunchy and satisfying trail mix.

Dessert: Mango and Coconut Chia Popsicles

Ingredients:
- Chia seeds
- Coconut milk
- Mango
- Honey

Nutritional Components (per serving):
- Protein: 6g
- Fiber: 8g

- Healthy Fats: 10g

Instructions:

- Mix chia seeds with coconut milk and let it sit in the refrigerator until it thickens.
- Blend mango with honey.
- Layer the chia mixture and mango puree in popsicle molds.
- Freeze until solid for a tropical and healthy popsicle treat.

Grocery List for Day 4:

Whole-grain tortilla, Eggs, Avocado, Cherry tomatoes, Salsa, Cilantro, Quinoa, Fresh mozzarella, Fresh basil, Balsamic glaze, Olive oil, Brown rice, Cucumber, Edamame, Seaweed sheets, Sesame seeds, Green onions, Almonds, Walnuts, Dried cranberries, Dark chocolate chips, Chia seeds, Coconut milk, Mango, Honey.

Day 5: Culinary Celebration

Breakfast: Blueberry and Almond Butter Smoothie Bowl

Ingredients:

- Blueberries
- Almond butter

- Almond milk
- Greek yogurt
- Granola
- Almonds (sliced)

Nutritional Components (per serving):
- Protein: 12g
- Fiber: 8g
- Healthy Fats: 10g

Instructions:
- Blend blueberries, almond butter, almond milk, and Greek yogurt until smooth.
- Pour into a bowl and top with granola and sliced almonds for a nutritious and delicious smoothie bowl.

Lunch: Mediterranean Chickpea Salad

Ingredients:
- Chickpeas (canned, drained, and rinsed)
- Cucumber
- Cherry tomatoes
- Red onion
- Kalamata olives
- Feta cheese
- Olive oil
- Lemon juice
- Oregano

- Salt and pepper to taste

Nutritional Components (per serving):
- Protein: 14g
- Fiber: 10g
- Healthy Fats: 12g

Instructions:
- Combine chickpeas with diced cucumber, halved cherry tomatoes, diced red onion, sliced Kalamata olives, and crumbled feta cheese.
- Drizzle with olive oil, lemon juice, sprinkle with oregano, salt, and pepper for a refreshing Mediterranean chickpea salad.

Dinner: Grilled Vegetable and Quinoa Stuffed Bell Peppers

Ingredients:
- Bell peppers (assorted colors)
- Quinoa
- Zucchini
- Eggplant
- Red onion
- Cherry tomatoes
- Olive oil
- Balsamic glaze
- Fresh basil

- Salt and pepper to taste

Nutritional Components (per serving):
- Protein: 12g
- Fiber: 8g
- Healthy Fats: 8g

Instructions:
- Cook quinoa according to package instructions.
- Slice zucchini, eggplant, red onion, and cherry tomatoes.
- Grill vegetables until tender.
- Mix grilled vegetables with cooked quinoa.
- Stuff bell peppers with the quinoa and vegetable mixture.
- Drizzle with olive oil, balsamic glaze, and sprinkle with fresh basil, salt, and pepper.

Snack: Greek Yogurt and Berry Parfait

Ingredients:
- Greek yogurt
- Mixed berries (strawberries, blueberries, raspberries)
- Honey
- Granola

Nutritional Components (per serving):
- Protein: 14g
- Fiber: 6g
- Healthy Fats: 8g

Instructions:
- Layer Greek yogurt with mixed berries, a drizzle of honey, and granola for a delightful and protein-rich snack.

Dessert: Dark Chocolate-Dipped Banana Bites

Ingredients:
- Banana
- Dark chocolate (70% cocoa or higher)
- Almonds (chopped)

Nutritional Components (per serving):
- Fiber: 5g
- Antioxidants: High

Instructions:
- Slice the banana into bite-sized pieces.
- Dip each piece into melted dark chocolate.
- Sprinkle with chopped almonds and let them cool until the chocolate hardens for a sweet and satisfying dessert.

Grocery List for Day 5:

Blueberries, Almond butter, Almond milk,Greek yogurt, Granola, Almonds (sliced), Chickpeas (canned), Cucumber, Cherry tomatoes, Red onion, Kalamata olives, Feta cheese, Olive oil, Lemon juice, Oregano, Salt, Pepper, Bell peppers (assorted colors), Quinoa, Zucchini, Eggplant, Cherry tomatoes, Balsamic glaze, Fresh basil, Dark chocolate (70% cocoa or higher), Banana, Almonds (chopped).

Day 6: Culinary Celebration

Breakfast: Berry and Spinach Smoothie

Ingredients:
- Mixed berries (strawberries, blueberries, raspberries)
- Spinach
- Greek yogurt
- Almond milk
- Chia seeds

Nutritional Components (per serving):
- Protein: 10g
- Fiber: 8g
- Healthy Fats: 8g

Instructions:
- Blend mixed berries, spinach, Greek yogurt, almond milk, and chia seeds until smooth.
- Enjoy a nutrient-packed and refreshing smoothie to kickstart your day.

Lunch: Quinoa and Avocado Salad

Ingredients:
- Quinoa
- Avocado
- Black beans (canned, drained, and rinsed)
- Corn kernels
- Cherry tomatoes
- Red onion
- Cilantro
- Lime
- Olive oil
- Salt and pepper to taste

Nutritional Components (per serving):
- Protein: 12g
- Fiber: 10g
- Healthy Fats: 15g
- Vitamin C: 25% of daily value

Instructions:

- Cook quinoa according to package instructions.
- Mix cooked quinoa with diced avocado, black beans, corn kernels, halved cherry tomatoes, diced red onion, chopped cilantro, a squeeze of lime juice, and olive oil.
- Season with salt and pepper for a vibrant and satisfying salad.

Dinner: Lemon Herb Baked Cod with Roasted Vegetables

Ingredients:

- Cod filets
- Lemon
- Fresh parsley
- Garlic
- Olive oil
- Sweet potatoes
- Broccoli
- Carrots
- Salt and pepper to taste

Nutritional Components (per serving):

- Protein: 20g
- Fiber: 8g
- Healthy Fats: 10g
- Vitamin A: 120% of daily value

Instructions:
- Preheat the oven and marinate cod filets in a mixture of lemon juice, chopped fresh parsley, minced garlic, and olive oil.
- Bake until the cod is cooked through.
- Roast sweet potatoes, broccoli, and carrots with olive oil, salt, and pepper.
- Serve the baked cod over a bed of roasted vegetables for a light and flavorful dinner.

Snack: Almond and Banana Rice Cake

Ingredients:
- Rice cakes
- Almond butter
- Banana

Nutritional Components (per serving):
- Protein: 6g
- Fiber: 4g
- Healthy Fats: 8g

Instructions:
- Spread almond butter on rice cakes and top with sliced banana for a crunchy and satisfying snack.

Dessert: Mixed Berry and Yogurt Popsicles

Ingredients:
- Mixed berries (strawberries, blueberries, raspberries)
- Greek yogurt
- Honey

Nutritional Components (per serving):
- Protein: 8g
- Fiber: 6g
- Healthy Fats: 6g

Instructions:
- Blend mixed berries, Greek yogurt, and honey until smooth.
- Pour into popsicle molds and freeze until solid for a cool and healthy dessert.

Grocery List for Day 6:
Mixed berries (strawberries, blueberries, raspberries), Spinach, Greek yogurt, Almond milk, Chia seeds, Quinoa, Avocado, Black beans (canned), Corn kernels, Cherry tomatoes, Red onion, Cilantro, Lime, Olive oil, Cod fillets, Lemon, Fresh parsley, Garlic, Sweet potatoes, Broccoli, Carrots, Rice cakes, Almond butter, Banana, Mixed berries (strawberries, blueberries, raspberries), Greek yogurt, Honey.

Day 7: Fiesta Fiesta!

Breakfast: Fiesta Scramble

Ingredients:
- Eggs
- Black beans (canned, drained, and rinsed)
- Bell peppers (assorted colors)
- Red onion
- Cherry tomatoes
- Avocado
- Cilantro
- Lime
- Salt and pepper to taste

Nutritional Components (per serving):
- Protein: 14g
- Fiber: 8g
- Healthy Fats: 10g
- Vitamin C: 60% of daily value

Instructions:
- Scramble eggs and mix in black beans, diced bell peppers, diced red onion, halved cherry tomatoes, sliced avocado, chopped cilantro, a squeeze of lime juice, salt, and pepper.
- Enjoy a festive and protein-rich scramble for a vibrant breakfast.

Lunch: Chicken and Vegetable Fajita Bowl

Ingredients:
- Chicken breast
- Bell peppers (assorted colors)
- Red onion
- Avocado
- Brown rice
- Black beans (canned, drained, and rinsed)
- Salsa
- Lime
- Cilantro
- Olive oil
- Fajita seasoning

Nutritional Components (per serving):
- Protein: 18g
- Fiber: 10g
- Healthy Fats: 10g
- Vitamin C: 150% of daily value

Instructions:
- Slice chicken breast, bell peppers, and red onion.
- Sauté in olive oil with fajita seasoning until cooked through.

- Serve over brown rice with black beans, sliced avocado, salsa, chopped cilantro, and a squeeze of lime for a flavorful fajita bowl.

Dinner: Shrimp and Mango Salsa Lettuce Wraps

Ingredients:
- Shrimp
- Lettuce leaves
- Mango
- Red bell pepper
- Red onion
- Cilantro
- Lime
- Olive oil
- Salt and pepper to taste

Nutritional Components (per serving):
- Protein: 20g
- Fiber: 6g
- Healthy Fats: 8g
- Vitamin C: 70% of daily value

Instructions:
- Grill shrimp until cooked.
- Prepare a salsa with diced mango, diced red bell pepper, diced red onion, chopped cilantro, a squeeze of lime, olive oil, salt, and pepper.

- Fill lettuce leaves with grilled shrimp and mango salsa for light and refreshing lettuce wraps.

Snack: Hummus and Veggie Sticks

Ingredients:
- Hummus
- Carrot sticks
- Cucumber sticks
- Bell pepper strips

Nutritional Components (per serving):
- Protein: 6g
- Fiber: 8g
- Healthy Fats: 8g

Instructions:
- Dip carrot sticks, cucumber sticks, and bell pepper strips into hummus for a satisfying and nutritious snack.

Dessert: Pineapple and Coconut Chia Pudding

Ingredients:
- Chia seeds
- Coconut milk
- Fresh pineapple
- Shredded coconut

Nutritional Components (per serving):
- Protein: 6g
- Fiber: 8g
- Healthy Fats: 10g

Instructions:
- Mix chia seeds with coconut milk and let it sit in the refrigerator until it thickens.
- Layer the chia mixture with fresh pineapple chunks and top with shredded coconut for a tropical and healthy chia pudding.

Grocery List for Day 7:

Eggs, Black beans (canned), Bell peppers (assorted colors), Red onion, Cherry tomatoes, Avocado, Cilantro, Lime, Salt, Pepper, Chicken breast, Brown rice, Salsa, Olive oil, Fajita seasoning, Lettuce leaves, Shrimp, Mango, Red bell pepper, Hummus, Carrot sticks, Cucumber sticks, Bell pepper strips, Chia seeds, Coconut milk, Fresh pineapple, Shredded coconut.

Congratulations on reaching Day 42 of your meal plan! I hope you've enjoyed the variety of flavors and nutrient-packed meals. Feel free to make any adjustments or let me know if you have specific preferences or dietary restrictions. Keep up the fantastic work on your journey to healthy eating!

CONCLUSION

Congratulations on completing this exciting 42-day journey with flavorful and nutritious meals! You've embraced the art of DASH diet meal prep, creating a symphony of tastes that dance on your palate while nourishing your body. As you savor the joy of vibrant ingredients and convenient containerized delights, remember that healthy eating is a journey, not a destination.

Let this be a launchpad for a sustainable and delicious lifestyle. The DASH diet, coupled with the convenience of meal prep containers, empowers you to make health-conscious choices without compromising on taste. Keep experimenting, keep enjoying, and most importantly, keep savoring the benefits of a well-nourished life.

As you savor each bite, know that you're investing in your well-being. Here's to more vibrant meals, endless possibilities, and a future filled with good health and great flavors. Cheers to you, the master chef of your DASH diet adventure!

May your culinary journey continue to be filled with delightful discoveries, nourishing your body and uplifting your spirits. Remember, every meal is an opportunity to celebrate your commitment to a healthier, happier you.

In the rhythmic dance of flavors and the colorful palette of ingredients, find joy and satisfaction. Let each meal be a reminder of the positive choices you've made and the well-deserved benefits you're reaping. With the DASH diet as your compass and meal prep as your ally, you're not just eating; you're savoring a lifestyle that embraces both health and happiness.

So, here's to more delicious chapters, more vibrant recipes, and more moments of culinary bliss. Keep savoring the journey, one meal at a time, and relish the goodness that comes from taking care of yourself. Your taste buds and your body will thank you. Bon appétit to a healthier, tastier you!